WITHDRAWN

D1362307

Recent Titles in
Health and Medical Issues Today

Medicare
Jennie Jacobs Kronenfeld

Illicit Drugs
Richard E. Isralowitz and Peter L. Myers

Animal-Assisted Therapy
Donald Altschiller

Alcohol
Peter L. Myers and Richard E. Isralowitz

Geriatrics
Carol Leth Stone

Plastic Surgery
Lana Thompson

Birth Control
Aharon W. Zorea

Bullying
Sally Kuykendall, PhD

Steroids
Aharon W. Zorea

Suicide and Mental Health
Rudy Nydegger

Cutting and Self-Harm
Chris Simpson

Discrimination against the Mentally Ill
Monica A. Joseph

Concussions
William Paul Meehan III

Drug Resistance
Sarah E. Boslaugh

Work-Life Balance
Janice Arenofsky

THE BODY SIZE AND HEALTH DEBATE

Christine L. B. Selby

Health and Medical Issues Today

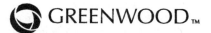

An Imprint of ABC-CLIO, LLC
Santa Barbara, California • Denver, Colorado

Copyright © 2017 by ABC-CLIO, LLC

All rights reserved. No part of this publication may be reproduced, stored in a retrieval system, or transmitted, in any form or by any means, electronic, mechanical, photocopying, recording, or otherwise, except for the inclusion of brief quotations in a review, without prior permission in writing from the publisher.

Library of Congress Cataloging-in-Publication Data

Names: Selby, Christine L. B., author.
Title: The body size and health debate / Christine L.B. Selby.
Description: Santa Barbara, California : Greenwood, [2017] | Series: Health and medical
    issues today | Includes bibliographical references and index.
Identifiers: LCCN 2017027840 (print) | LCCN 2017029383 (ebook) |
    ISBN 9781440848063 (ebook) | ISBN 9781440848056 (alk. paper)
Subjects: | MESH: Body Weight | Obesity—complications | Obesity—psychology |
    Social Perception | Body Image–psychology | Healthy Lifestyle | United States
Classification: LCC RA645.O23 (ebook) | LCC RA645.O23 (print) | NLM WD 210 |
    DDC 362.1963/98—dc23
LC record available at https://lccn.loc.gov/2017027840

ISBN: 978-1-4408-4805-6 (print)
      978-1-4408-4806-3 (ebook)

21 20 19 18 17   1 2 3 4 5

This book is also available as an eBook.

Greenwood
An Imprint of ABC-CLIO, LLC

ABC-CLIO, LLC
130 Cremona Drive, P.O. Box 1911
Santa Barbara, California 93116–1911
www.abc-clio.com

This book is printed on acid-free paper ∞

Manufactured in the United States of America

This book discusses treatments (including types of medication and mental health therapies), diagnostic tests for various symptoms and mental health disorders, and organizations. The authors have made every effort to present accurate and up-to-date information. However, the information in this book is not intended to recommend or endorse particular treatments or organizations, or substitute for the care or medical advice of a qualified health professional, or used to alter any medical therapy without a medical doctor's advice. Specific situations may require specific therapeutic approaches not included in this book. For those reasons, we recommend that readers follow the advice of qualified health care professionals directly involved in their care. Readers who suspect they may have specific medical problems should consult a physician about any suggestions made in this book.

This book is dedicated to those who struggle with accepting their body as it is no matter its weight, shape, or size.

CONTENTS

Series Foreword   ix

Preface   xi

Acknowledgments   xv

Part I: Overview of the Body Size and Health Debate   **1**

1   Changing Shape of the Ideal Body throughout
    the 20th Century   3

2   Health and Body Mass Index (BMI)   21

3   Rates of Obesity and Targeted Prevention Efforts   41

4   Consequences of How Overweight and Obese Are
    Treated and Viewed by Society   65

5   Health at Every Size®   87

Part II: Controversies and Issues   **97**

6   Body Image and Happiness: Should We Be Focused on
    Body Shape and Size?   99

7   Can Overweight or Obese Bodies Really Be Healthy?   109

8   Is Personal Choice a Relevant Argument for Body Size?   133

9   Applications of Health at Every Size®   149

Part III: Scenarios   **163**

Case Illustrations   165

Glossary   179
Timeline   183
Sources for Further Information   187
Bibliography   191
Index   201
About the Author   209

SERIES FOREWORD

Every day, the public is bombarded with information on developments in medicine and health care. Whether it is on the latest techniques in treatment or research, or on concerns over public health threats, this information directly affects the lives of people more than almost any other issue. Although there are many sources for understanding these topics—from websites and blogs to newspapers and magazines—students and ordinary citizens often need one resource that makes sense of the complex health and medical issues affecting their daily lives.

The *Health and Medical Issues Today* series provides just such a one-stop resource for obtaining a solid overview of the most controversial areas of health care in the 21st century. Each volume addresses one topic and provides a balanced summary of what is known. These volumes provide an excellent first step for students and lay people interested in understanding how health care works in our society today.

Each volume is broken into several sections to provide readers and researchers with easy access to the information they need:

> Section I provides overview chapters on background information—including chapters on such areas as the historical, scientific, medical, social, and legal issues involved—that a citizen needs to intelligently understand the topic.
> Section II provides capsule examinations of the most heated contemporary issues and debates, and analyzes in a balanced manner the viewpoints held by various advocates in the debates.
> Section III provides case studies that show examples of the concepts discussed in the previous sections.

A selection of reference material, such as a timeline of important events, a directory of organizations, a glossary, and a bibliography, serve as the best next step in learning about the topic at hand.

The *Health and Medical Issues Today* series strives to provide readers with all the information needed to begin making sense of some of the most important debates going on in the world today. The series includes volumes on such topics as stem-cell research, obesity, gene therapy, alternative medicine, organ transplantation, mental health, and more.

PREFACE

The Body Size and Health Debate is part of the *Health and Medical Issues Today* series. This book is of particular interest for those who want to develop a better understanding of how body size and health are viewed in the United States. Although the United States is not alone in its focus on a particular version of attractiveness for both females and males, there is a clear message in this country that being overweight or obese is not only unattractive but also decidedly unhealthy. This book is, in many ways, a labor of love. I routinely work with men and women who struggle with body image issues as well as the pressure they feel from nearly everywhere to lose weight. Many are also told unequivocally that they cannot be healthy unless they do lose weight. There remains a healthy and at times highly contentious debate among health-care providers about whether or not someone can be healthy even if their body mass index (BMI) places them in the range of obesity. My hope is that after reading this book you will learn about research yielding results that are new to you and that you are provided with enough information that you will learn more about these issues and come to your own, well-thought-out and fully informed conclusion.

As already noted, this book covers information related to body weight, shape, and size explicitly as well as the degree to which body size reveals anything about our health status. The book is organized into three parts. Part I includes several chapters on topics ranging from what is considered to be the ideal body to an approach to weight and health that is controversial. Chapter 1 explores the expectations for the ideal body shape and size throughout modern history. Emphasis is on expectations for women's bodies; however, expectations for males are explored as well. Chapter 2 examines how health is defined, how health is often measured by body weight and size, and the veracity of using such a measure as a barometer of health. The focus of Chapter 3 turns to the rates of obesity in the United States and efforts designed to prevent obesity particularly in children; Chapter 4 examines the effects that these efforts and other factors have on the physical and psychological wellbeing of those with larger bodies. Finally, Chapter 5 introduces readers to an approach to health and weight that is controversial: the Health at Every Size® approach. The chapter also examines evidence suggesting that the approach has merit as well as concerns about whether or not the approach is safe.

Part II includes individual chapters exploring a different controversy. The first controversy covered in Chapter 6 involves the connection between body image and happiness and whether or not trying to achieve the ideal body will lead to overall life satisfaction. Chapter 7 examines the controversy of whether or not someone with an obese body can be healthy by reviewing the diseases connected with obesity, why some question this connection, and if weight loss is the answer, whether or not weight loss is truly possible. Chapter 8 focuses on the issues of personal choice and personal responsibility, and what role those play in whether or not each of us owes having a normal body size to society at large. Finally, Chapter 9 examines how the Health at Every Size® approach can be applied to various settings and services. Since this approach is, in and of itself, controversial, applying the approach to schools, healthcare, and other public services can be viewed as controversial as well.

Part III includes five different scenarios involving weight, weight loss, and health followed by an analysis of the scenario. Readers are presented with a description of various situations that occur in real life and how they can be handled first from the mainstream perspective and then from the Health at Every Size® perspective. The first scenario describes an elementary school aged boy who has received a BMI report card from his school. Scenario two involves an 18-year-old female high school student who is attempting to achieve a more curvy body so she is more attractive to men she might date. Scenario three illustrates a 45-year-old male's struggle to maintain a normal weight and his subsequent decision to pursue weight loss surgery. Scenario four involves a young adult female's struggle to make sense of being told to lose weight by her primary care provider despite having test results showing she is healthy. Finally, scenario five describes a young woman's history of frustrating weight loss efforts which have led her to decide to focus on her health instead of her weight.

Finally, this book includes a resource section containing both online and print sources, a timeline of important events involving body size and/

or health, a glossary of terms that may be unfamiliar to readers, and a bibliography of sources from which information included in this book was gleaned.

I hope you enjoy learning about the debate that exists regarding body size and health including reading about current research that may challenge some long-standing beliefs.

ACKNOWLEDGMENTS

Completing this project could not have been accomplished without a great deal of support. First and foremost, I would like to thank my family: my husband and my two boys. Their support for this project allowed me to take the time and energy I needed to complete this book and make it something I can be proud of. I would also like to thank my psychology colleagues at Husson University in Bangor, Maine, who endured my lack of availability particularly for weekly lunch get-togethers, and for having my office door closed more than usual. This is the second book project that I have worked on with Maxine Taylor at ABC-CLIO. As always she was supportive of my work, was tolerant of minor delays, and provided invaluable feedback on the structure and organization of the content. This book is in the form it is because of her excellent guidance. Finally, I would like to thank my parents for their support. Although my mom did not live to see the publication of this book, both she and my father instilled in me an appreciation for the written word and quite frankly did not stand in my way as I pursued my desires in both my personal life and my career.

PART I

Overview of the Body Size and Health Debate

Changing Shape of the Ideal Body throughout the 20th Century

Many readers undoubtedly know the ideal shape and size of a woman's body has changed throughout history. From the voluptuous figure of the Renaissance woman to the thin but curvy body of the 21st century, as long as there has been graphic representation of the human form there has been a body ideal. Most attention has historically been paid to the female form largely due to the fact that a woman's appearance is thought to be her most valuable asset; however, males have a standard to meet as well.

The sections that follow primarily take a look at what the ideal female body has been during the 20th century and into the 21st century. To best understand and offer a context as to why a particular body type was prized, each time period includes a brief overview of the significant events and attitudes of that time. The male body, too, has been scrutinized over the years, but much less is written about the pressures men feel to achieve a particular look—though in recent years there seems to be more of an acknowledgment by researchers and the public that males, too, are held to an impossibly high standard. A single section takes a brief look at the pressures males have and continue to experience. This chapter culminates in examining the current ideal for both males and females as well as the impact these unrealistic standards have on both physical and mental health.

FEMALES: LATE 1800s AND EARLY 1900s

In the late 1800s and into the early 1900s, women did not yet have the right to vote. This was, however, the era of the suffragists, and on

June 4, 1919, Congress passed the 19th Amendment, which was ultimately ratified on August 18, 1920. Although women were starting to speak up and given some important responsibilities, during this time women were believed to be incapable of performing outside of the home. It was thought that should they be allowed to hold formal positions in business or government they might be a threat to the stability of the economy and the country. In fact, physicians of the day advised young women against going to college (which would, of course, make them better prepared for the business world), as it was thought to be dangerous to a woman's health since the stress of studying and thinking would damage her reproductive capabilities. Not only men, but many women were on board with leaving things the way they were. Society depended on men and women remaining in their traditional roles.

One element of society during this era was polite society—a term referring to the wealthy elite of the time and their extravagant social gatherings. Women were in charge of these events—the men made the money to fund them. Women wore full-length dresses that dragged across the ground and collars that stopped just below one's chin. Even swimming required the body to be fully covered in heavy material preventing actual swimming—all they could do was float. A woman's body was to be covered up. Anything remotely referring to sex or the sexuality of women was strictly prohibited. In fact, in 1873, a law called the 1873 Comstock Law was enacted, which outlawed the distribution of anything indecent or salacious, including materials that included information about birth control.

In the early 1900s, magazines soared in popularity; among them was the *Ladies' Home Journal*. This and other magazines marketed to women included stories and cartoons thought to tap into what women of that era wanted to read and look at. These periodicals also included "fashion plates," which referred to the printing practice of using engravings that had color applied to them by hand. Thus, the women depicted in these images were referred to as fashion plates. Charles Dana Gibson was an artist whose works were widely printed and published in women's magazines, often on the cover. His renderings of women wearing the latest fashions of the period captured not only the fashion itself but also the ideal silhouette and accompanying attitude. The Gibson Girl, the moniker given to his depictions, portrayed women as not only fashionable but aloof and sophisticated. This was a divergence from the nurturing and gentle image many people had of women.

The Gibson Girl's typical look involved long hair arranged on top of her head in a chignon. She wore a high-collared shirtwaist, which was a shirt gathered at the waist no doubt to enhance that part of the body, and a skirt.

The Gibson Girl was curvy; however, this silhouette was not achieved naturally. Corsets were a staple in a proper woman's wardrobe, and the swan-bill corset helped women achieve the Gibson Girl look: heavily cinched at the waist resulting in the hourglass shape of much fuller bust and hips. Women were so taken by this look that some were willing to do whatever it took to achieve it. Anna Held, a showgirl of the time, desired the Gibson Girl silhouette so much that she had a rib surgically removed to achieve an 18-inch waist. By 1910, Gibson's depictions of the ideal woman gave way to Fisher Girls, Christy Girls, and Brinkley Girls, each named after their artist-creators.

Fisher Girls were portrayed as more child-like than the Gibson Girl. The Fisher Girls appeared to be younger and more playful and naive rather than worldly. Both the Fisher illustrations and the Christy Girls images depicted girls who were engaged in physical activity and thus had a more athletic appearance. The Brinkley Girl, named after Nell Brinkley, the only women artist in this context, was commissioned by publishing mogul William Randolph Hearst to produce images of women not based on whom one might see on a day-to-day basis, but a romanticized version of women. Despite this request, Brinkley's girl reflected what the suffragists were fighting for: independence and freedom. Brinkley Girls were not constrained by corsets or swim caps, and like the Fisher and Christy Girls, they, too, were depicted engaged in some activity rather than simply striking a pose.

Women's fashion changed to reflect the changes in women's lives. Women desired to do away with the constraints of corseted waists and long, heavy dresses so that they could be more comfortable and wear clothing that was more practical. The introduction of the shirtwaist to women's fashion was one such indicator as was the shortening of women's skirts so that they could move comfortably or ride a bicycle safely. The end of this time period was marked by World War I—the Great War as it was known then. The thousands of men fighting overseas meant that an equal number of jobs were now vacant. Women quickly filled those positions, not just to be sure the work was done, but because they needed an income since their husbands, fathers, and brothers were no longer at home earning a wage.

FEMALES: 1920s

The Flapper was the iconic image of the 1920s, and one of the events that helped define this era was the ratification of the 19th Amendment in 1920: women's right to vote. During the same year, Congress created the Women's Bureau in the Department of Labor in an effort to protect women in the workforce. Prior to 1920 was the Great War—World War I, which meant that the women during the era of the Great War filled the jobs of the men who went off to fight, many of whom never returned. Working women started to become more commonplace. Despite the necessity of work, men and women alike viewed women's employment as temporary, as they were not really embarking on careers. As such, women earned far less than their male counterparts. Popular magazines of the day continued to remind girls and women that they were socially and biologically predisposed to engage in domestic duties. They admonished anything that took them away from their traditional roles and that would contribute to their "failure" as future mothers and wives. The message was clear: do not work.

Fashion prior to the 1920s was designed to hide how women's bodies naturally looked by using metal and bone corsets to artificially produced an hourglass shape and to improve one's figure. The voluminous use of fabric helped to hide anything that might be considered unappealing. The fashion of the 1920s by contrast was not designed to intentionally hide or enhance the female body; however, women with larger bodies may have used various forms of binding to flatten their breasts since the Flapper look was sleek, thin, and flat chested.

This change in fashion was not an easy transition. Resistance to getting rid of corsets and the like was expressed via advertisements that communicated the perils of not wearing these items by using racist language and images imploring well-to-do white women not do away with this necessary garment. Corsets were also marketed directly to women whose bodies changed as a result of bearing children, and corset manufacturer preyed on women's fear of aging and disease by claiming that corsets would help you stay youthful and keep you from getting ill. Getting rid of such undergarments and aspiring to the thinner look of the Flapper—which did not require the female form to be squeezed or to make other parts of one's anatomy appear larger—meant that there was greater emphasis on how the female body looked naturally. This also meant that there was nothing to hide behind and women became aware of their weight in a way they had not before. Women of the 1920s became invested in making sure they were small enough to fit this new, sleek image which meant they were dieting.

Prior to the 1920s, larger bodies were viewed as a sign of prosperity. A larger body meant greater resources and hearty food. Meal times were events with multiple courses including more than one type of meat, multiple starches, and myriad desserts. By the 1920s, however, families were shrinking the size of their menus including what was on them. This changed in part due to the invention of many kitchen appliances, but there was also a shift to the idea that larger bodies were unhealthier than thinner ones. Thus, smaller meals were consumed along with more fruits and vegetables.

Lulu Hunt Peters, a physician, may well have been the first weight loss doctor. In 1923, she published a book entitled *Diet and Health, with Key to the Calories*, which quickly became a best seller and remained a best seller for four years. She promised to "save" women from being fat so that they were no longer the subject of ridicule. She took a scientific approach to weight loss focusing on calories consumed and calories burned and warned her readers and patients against taking pills or other medication that promised to help women lose weight. She also warned that a woman embarking on a weight loss journey would be sabotaged in her attempts to lose weight by her husband, who did not like thin women and family and friends who were convinced that a larger body was a healthier body, and that losing weight would put her at risk for serious illness and death.

An additional factor contributing to women's awareness of their weight was the mass manufacturing of clothes. Prior to the 1920s, women constructed their own clothes to fit or had a seamstress custom fit their wardrobe. After the Great War, clothing manufacturers created standardized sizing which meant that each size had specific measurements. This, of course, made it much easier for manufacturers to mass produce clothing quickly. The problem for the consumer, of course, was that her body had to fit into one of these predetermined sizes.

The emphasis on female appearance was not limited to her shape and size. She was also more aware than ever of how her skin and face looked. Women began carrying compact mirrors with them so that they could make sure their makeup and overall appearance was still "acceptable." Print media was marketing to women's fears that if she was not attractive and youthful enough then a man would not want to be with her let alone touch her. This was the era of cosmetic empires such as Maybelline and Elizabeth Arden, which helped to normalize the use of makeup (prior to this time was reserved for stage performers), and the designer Coco Chanel, whose fashion house continues to influence clothing design and fragrance trends in the 21st century.

The issue of beauty with respect to race revealed a decidedly Caucasian-centric view of beauty. Madame E. Azalia Hackley was a renowned soprano and African American woman. She took issue with an article that appeared in 1920 describing what a beautiful woman looks like. She noted that the emphasis was entirely on white skin and the physical features of white women. She took it upon herself to speak out about how women can be beautiful no matter their racial background and that true beauty comes from within.

FEMALES: 1930s AND 1940s

The 1930s and 1940s in the United States are most often thought of in terms of the stock market crash and the Great Depression that immediately followed. The 1940s are also remembered as the time in history that saw the second Great War: World War II. Both events had a significant impact on women not only in terms of how they lived their lives and what they were "allowed" to do, but also in terms of fashion. During this era, Amelia Earhart took flight, Ella Fitzgerald began her singing career, and Eleanor Roosevelt fought for the fair treatment of women. These trailblazing women helped to redefine what women are capable of and how they should expect to be treated.

The stock market crash in 1929 resulted in a great deal of personal and economic turmoil. Many people lived in abject poverty because they lost everything including their jobs. Most could not find new employment. As a result, women were strongly discouraged to even consider entering the workforce. The message was clear: because jobs are scarce, you do not belong in the workplace and should refocus your energies on the home. Some even blamed women being in the workforce to begin with as the cause of the Great Depression. This, of course, was untrue but reflected the view of working women at the time.

Betty Boop was introduced to the world in the 1930s. She was the first cartoon character that exhibited sexuality. She wore a short strapless dress, high heels, and a visible garter. She wore jewelry and had large eyes with pronounced eye lashes. She was often depicted as the object of male attention but remained a character that displayed innocence and a child-like quality. In short, she portrayed women as innocent but sexual. The burgeoning display of female sexuality on the printed page or on the silver screen created a great deal of discomfort for a lot of people of the day. Whether it had to do with what women could and could not show of their bodies or what types of scenarios were depicted on screen, the *Hays Code of the 1930s* regulated proper and moral behavior shown in film.

The 1920s saw a firm shift away from internal beauty to external beauty. Makeup became more acceptable and was associated with the average woman rather than solely women with "loose morals." When the 1930s rolled around mass advertising had understood the shift and began marketing beauty products to all women. Women were told that they needed the cosmetics in order to avoid looking old or enduring the pain of social isolation as a result of not looking good enough. They peddled the idea that looking your best meant that you would have friends, could get and keep a husband, and could still look young, which was clearly more desirable than looking old. Prior advertisements encouraged women to dress and look a certain way to please themselves, whereas now the messages were that you should care what other people think.

Coinciding with the shift to external beauty was a change in fashion in the 1930s. Women's skirt lengths dropped to cover more of the legs placing emphasis on the ankles, and the waistline was raised to highlight a woman's natural curves. The realities of the Great Depression, however, meant that materials were scarce and expensive, so being frugal was necessary. This meant that a more tailored look began to dominate women's fashion, which further accentuated the shape and size of a woman's body. At the same time, however, highly athletic women were starting to gain notoriety. This caused some concern and confusion among those who could only picture women wearing "proper" clothing and being engaged in domestic activities—not displaying their strength or prowess in a sporting arena. A stronger, more capable woman would soon make an appearance in the 1940s.

When the United States officially entered World War II, thousands of men were shipped off to war, which left many vacancies. In order to keep up with the demands of war, many new jobs were created but without men to fill them. Women were by and large the only ones around to fill these positions, which they did proudly and effectively. As a result, Rosie the Riveter was born.

Rosie was contrived by the Office of War Information (OWI) whose purpose was to make sure everyone played their part in the war by continuing to be smart and frugal. Women were once again targeted as they were the ones running the home and needed to be made aware of the importance of rationing food and reusing materials when possible. The OWI was also tasked with recruiting women to help with the war effort directly. The marketing sent the message that women could join the fight and thereby support their male loved ones. Additionally, the print campaign initially depicted women not as hardworking or strong but as feminine and attractive. Rosie the Riveter, a physically strong woman, dressed for hard labor was introduced just prior to Pearl Harbor. Despite her fierce appearance, she was still depicted with makeup, and her story was that she was not only working but still doing the important work of keeping the home fires burning—she took care of her children, made the home comfortable, and had well-prepared meals. In short, Rosie the Riveter did it all. This brought into awareness the challenges of doing a lot. Women on the job were more likely to ask for more time off than their male counterparts because they were also juggling the demands of childcare. Eventually, however, Rosie the Riveter gave way to Rosie the Pinup Girl. These were print images of starlets wearing a svelte evening gown or a revealing bathing suit and were distributed to men fighting in the war.

FEMALES: 1950s AND 1960s

Margaret Chase Smith, a senator from Maine and the first woman to be elected to the U.S. Senate, took on Senator Joseph McCarthy of Wisconsin regarding his relentless pursuit of rousting communists among American citizens. She not only challenged a powerful U.S. senator but also the fact that women could not be powerful in their own right. In 1955, Rosa Parks committed a criminal act when she refused to vacate her seat on a bus for a white person. In 1963, Martin Luther King Jr. gave his *I Have a Dream* speech in Washington, D.C., in front of the Lincoln Memorial. Activists began the fight for the rights of homosexuals. The fallout shelter was a cultural phenomenon, and the end of this era culminated in "one small step for man." Much happened in the 1950s and 1960s, not only for the country as a whole but for women in particular.

The 1950s was a wealthy decade. People including girls and young women had money to spend. Females influenced capitalism at the time by funneling their money to musicians they worshiped and fashions they liked. In doing so, they help to shape the culture. Despite this influence, there was still heavy pressure on girls to ensure they were date-able and marriage material. In order to be that, they had to be sure they looked just right, acted the right way, and above all had their life's ambition to be a homemaker. It was a woman's job to make sure married life and home life were enjoyable and satisfying for her husband. The 1950s was the decade of the MRS degree, which involved going to college for the express purpose of finding a suitable husband. Despite this continued mantra, by the end of the 1960s, women were much more likely to be found in the workplace engaged in a variety of vocations.

In 1959, the Barbie® doll was born. Even at that time, her shape and size were questioned, but she went to market in the form that would remain relatively unchanged for over 50 years. Barbie's shape and size has been questioned and debated since she was introduced to the world, but it was not until 2000 that Margo Maine determined that if Barbie® were a real person her proportions would be such that she would not be able to stand upright due to the weight of her chest and the size of her feet. She would have had to have ribs surgically removed due to the size of her waist, and she would more than likely be diagnosed with anorexia nervosa due to her low estimated body mass index. Regardless she remained a cultural icon and held a shape that many girls and young women aspired to achieve.

Prior to the production of the Barbie® doll, the feminine ideal was curvy. The sex symbols at that time were Marilyn Monroe, Betty Grable, and Lana Turner, all of whom boasted womanly curves. In the mid-1950s, things changed with the emergence of Audrey Hepburn. She was slim and not at all curvy. She was considered by some to be flat chested with a figure more like a boy's than a woman's. She was appealing to many women because she interpreted what it meant to be feminine in her own way. She dressed the way she wanted, cut her hair the way she wanted, and encouraged women to be themselves (though many ended up imitating her signature style). Audrey Hepburn's look may have paved the way for the icon of the following decade.

The mid-1960s celebrated a new feminine ideal when Leslie Hornsby hit the scene. She is most famously known as Twiggy. She was thin and petite showing off thin legs and arms. She was often described as having a boyish figure. She was not at all reminiscent of the 1950s' bombshells who sported the classic hourglass figure. Teenage girls and women tossed aside the trappings of the 1950s attire and clamored for miniskirts, pantyhose, and a bra that was not pointy (or no bra at all). Twiggy was reportedly not thin because she ate very little. She apparently tried to gain weight but could not and declared that she did not think she was attractive. This did not, however, prevent girls and women from trying to achieve her body shape and size. As a result, the quest to lose weight skyrocketed, and one of the most profitable weight loss companies ever launched started in 1963: Weight Watchers®.

FEMALES: 1970s TO 1990s

In the summer of 1970, the National Organization of Women organized a strike. Their meager membership numbers coordinated a national effort that encouraged women to walk out of their jobs for the day—whether the job was outside of the home and paid, or inside the home as a homemaker and unpaid. The result? Tens of thousands of women and men across the United States went on strike in an effort to protest the inequality that still existed between men and women despite laws that prohibited paying women less for doing equal work. Women were still held culturally captive to traditionally "female" roles. They continued to encounter too many hurdles when pursuing skills and passions that men pursued without thought to whether or not they would be allowed to.

Powerful women such as Gloria Steinem, an outspoken activist, Billy Jean King, a professional tennis player who beat Bobby Riggs in the "Battle of the Sexes" and won in straight sets, and Sally Ride, who was the first female astronaut to have a mission in space, demonstrated the power and tenacity that women were capable of. Women were taking on more diverse roles in the workforce, and by the late 1970s and 1980s, the fashions of the day in part reflected this movement. Clothing for women included outfits that mimicked elements of the man's business suit whether in terms of the type of fabric or how the garment was styled. These outfits were still decidedly feminine but reflected the idea that women needed to dress similar to their male counterparts to be taken seriously.

Despite the growing choices available, women were still concerned with their figures and how they looked. The 1980s and 1990s saw a new industry of diet food boom. More and more companies recognized the desire many women had to lose weight and scrambled to produce food products that could be identified as "diet" food, foods low in fat, or foods low in calories. Magazines consistently had stories about significantly overweight women and what they did to lose many pounds of weight. These magazines were consistently replete with workout plans or exercise apparatus "guaranteed" to slim one part of the body or another. In aggregate, this further reinforced the idea for women that they should be losing weight. One of the results of this cultural obsession with weight loss was a corresponding rise in eating disorders. They certainly existed prior to this time period, but it was not until the 1980s and 1990s that lay people and professionals alike recognized that eating disorders were problems and could be physically devastating and deadly.

During the 1970s to 1990s, formalized weight loss programs had franchises throughout the country and produced infomercials demonstrating the purpose and effectiveness of their products. Books on how to diet and lose weight became international best sellers, and diet pills were easily accessible at any drug or grocery store. In the 1980s, a relatively curvy yet still slim Cindy Crawford was the beauty ideal that was difficult for most women to emulate, but by the 1990s, an even more impossible standard was born known as the "heroin chic" look popularized by supermodel Kate Moss. As the standard of beauty, mannequins in department stores reflected this shift in body type. The mannequins manufactured to represent this new ideal were several inches taller than the average woman in the United States and weighed considerably less. The significant difference between what women were seeing in fashion magazines and clothing stores and their own bodies garnered attention from scientists interested in the impact this disparity may have on women.

Scientists in recent years have examined women's perceptions of themselves and their self-esteem. Not surprisingly, these studies revealed that while not all women categorized themselves as overweight, the vast majority of women believe they needed to lose some weight. Additionally, researchers examining the impact of print magazines aimed at women found that women experienced a measurable drop in self-esteem after 2–3 minutes of flipping through these magazines. Women were confronted by terms such as "thunder thighs" and "orange-peel skin" (i.e., cellulite), which were conditions that every woman should be wary of and take steps to correct should they notice these conditions affecting their own body.

Over the decades of the 20th century and into the 21st century, women have fought to have more rights as U.S. citizens and to have their talents and skills valued even if those talents did not involve being a wife and a mother. Great strides have been made in these efforts; however, running parallel to the quest for equality were messages about how to be sure women remained attractive—a commodity that is still thought to be a woman's greatest asset.

A LOOK AT MALE STANDARDS WITHIN THE 20TH CENTURY

Less has been written about the pressures and expectations boys and men face to achieve a particular ideal. It has been suggested that this may be because the pressure to conform is much greater for females, and that historically the ideal female body (at whatever time in history) is the most important thing a woman can work toward; she should be sure she looks "right" above all other pursuits. While it may be true that the pressure for females is more significant than it is for males, there is little doubt that boys and men have a standard too. As far back as Ancient Egypt, men have strived to address certain problem areas including hair loss. Historically, hair loss along with fitness level and sexual functioning have been the target areas that men have been consistently told are things they should pay close attention to in order to maintain their masculinity.

Hair Loss

Just as small hips, smooth skin, and a toned body have signified youthfulness in women, a full head of hair has been a sign of youth and vitality for men. Men are consistently told that if their hair is thinning (which happens to a fifth of all men by the age of 20), then there is something wrong with them and they need to fix it. In the modern era, men are shown via television and print ads that if they are able to prevent hair loss altogether or regrow lost hair then they will garner the affection of women— of course not just any women, but women who fit the female ideal standard

of beauty. Remedies for hair loss are not, however, just a modern phenomenon. Ancient Egyptians dealing with hair loss might have been prescribed a potion made out of the nail clippings of human beings and parts
of various animals including the ibex, crocodile, lion, and hedgehog.

Modern hair loss treatments have included chemical-based salves that
are applied directly to balding areas. These products were marketed to
those who already lost significant amounts of hair along with the promise
that the product would stimulate hair follicles to grow hair again. There
have been products in spray cans that when sprayed all over a man's head
seem to magically increase the thickness of existing hair thereby covering
the balding areas. And, of course, there has been a multitude of surgical
procedures involving transplanting donor hair, moving hair from one part
of the head to another, implanting hair directly into the scalp, and surgically implanting snaps so that a toupee could be attached and removed as
desired.

Being Physically Fit

Maintaining an active and fit body has long been an expectation for
men. Engaging in physical activity and achieving a "perfect" body was
thought to be a sign of heightened spirituality during the 1800s. The more
active and fit a male was, the less likely he was to engage in "immoral"
activities. Thus pursuing fitness was thought to not only benefit him but
also society at large. Over the decades, the purpose of physical activity has
changed and has included the development not only of strength and agility
but also sportsmanship, which was believed to benefit men in the business
world as sportsmanship promoted leadership abilities. The emphasis on
strength alone was prominent during the eras of boxing and weight lifting,
which was the precursor to body building. Weight lifting was designed to
display one's strength, whereas body building was designed to show off
one's aesthetic.

Despite this historic emphasis on lean and fit bodies, larger bodies due
to fat composition rather than muscle mass have not always been reviled.
The term gluttony was used in the mid-19th century to refer to those who
had larger bodies and who were thought to be at greater risk for health
problems. This body type was also thought to correlate with engaging in
excessive sexual behaviors which was considered immoral and thus unde-
sirable. By the late 19th century, however, during the country's Gilded
Age, fatter bodies were associated with being wealthier, while smaller
male bodies were associated with poverty. So, for a short period of time,
it was to a man's advantage to be overweight so that he could physically

manifest his degree of wealth. This acceptance of larger bodies was short-lived, as fitter and leaner bodies resurged as the ideal.

In the 1920s when Hollywood became home to the burgeoning motion picture industry, more people than ever before were exposed to bodies that had to look good on film. This meant they needed to be fit and lean since being on film artificially added many pounds to the appearance of one's body. Additionally, many actors were required to engage in physically demanding activities (e.g., horseback riding) making fitness a priority so that they could reliably complete these activities. Hollywood actors (both male and female) therefore were young, slim, and needed bodies that looked healthy and sexy on a large screen.

Two decades later, in the 1940s, psychologist William Sheldon developed a standard for three body types: ectomorph, mesomorph, and endomorph. These body types ranged from skinny to overweight, respectively. Sheldon also suggested that certain personality characteristics could be attributed to each body type, which still endure to this day. He characterized ectomorphs as being more intelligent than the other two types, but they were also prone to being nervous or anxious. On the other end of the spectrum was the endomorphs who were described as being warm and friendly, but also lazy and gluttonous. The middle body type, mesomorph, was characterized by strength, masculinity, and energy. There was virtually nothing negative about this body type. Sheldon's work reinforced the idea that a fitter body type was ideal not only in terms of how one looked but also in terms of one's personality. The major problem with Sheldon's work is that he based the descriptions of personality associated with each body type on pure conjecture. He did not have any scientific evidence to support his claims that if one's body type is known then his or her personality and behavior characteristics could also be known. His ideas suggested that all you had to do was look at someone and you would know a lot about what kind of person they were. Sheldon's claims were not that dissimilar to Franz Gall's phrenology, which suggested that the various bumps on your head could reveal your personality traits. The difference between these two ideas is that Gall's theory has been thoroughly debunked whereas Sheldon's ideas have endured.

Whether trying to ensure one is perceived as strong, energetic, and masculine, or trying to live up to the current ideal for attractiveness many men have elected to undergo cosmetic surgery to alter the size and shape of various aspects of the body. Cosmetic surgery for men has been documented as far back as the seventh century when some men had what is now known as rhinoplasty or a "nose job." Modern-day surgeries for men include nose jobs, liposuction, and implants to make various areas of the body appear larger and more muscular. In addition to surgery, men and adolescent boys may turn to steroids to ensure rapid and enhanced development of muscle mass. Regardless of the methods used to try to appear younger, more attractive, and more masculine, ultimately men are told they need to do whatever it takes to be attractive so that they can also display their sexual prowess.

Sexual Functioning

At various points in time, a positive view of male sexuality may have depended on his ability to function sexually or on whether he looked good enough for sex. Looking good for sex did not exclusively refer to how muscular he was, but it also referred to whether his penis and its functioning was adequate. *Impotence*, a term used to refer to the inability for a male to achieve an erection or for premature ejaculation, has been thought, without scientific basis, to have been an indicator of infertility, the result of masturbatory activity, or promiscuity. Regardless, the sexual functioning of a male has been and continues to be a source of power for men. If they are unable to perform as expected, then they are thought to be weak and less of a man. Or if they are able to perform but the appearance of their penis is unsatisfactory, their masculinity takes a significant hit.

The tendency to equate masculinity with sexuality helps to explain why many men use chemicals (prescription or otherwise) to ensure that they can perform, use pumps to temporarily enlarge the size of the penis, penile implants for the same purpose, or elect to have phalloplasty—a collection of surgical procedures intended to increase the length of the penis and/ or its girth. One surgeon, Melvyn Rosenstein, in the early to mid-1990s boasted that he collected $30 million performing these procedures and intended to make penis enlargement for men as commonplace as breast enlargement was for women. The Medical Board of the State of California, where many of these surgeries were performed, declared these procedures to be a danger to the public after multiple law suits were brought against the physician for men who were left disfigured or in tremendous pain as a result of the surgery.

There is little doubt that males have been held to standards of attractiveness that are as unrealistic and potentially harmful as the standards for women. The standards themselves are different but seem to communicate a similar message. If you want to be attractive to potential mates and if you want to be sure you are perceived as ultra-masculine or feminine, then you will learn about and adhere to the standards of attractiveness for your sex no matter the cost.

THIN IDEAL AND MUSCULAR IDEAL: THE CURRENT STANDARDS

The current ideals for male and female bodies have been termed the muscular ideal and the thin ideal, respectively. The thin ideal for female bodies is often described in terms of a skinny body with a small waist and low body fat. Others have suggested that the thin ideal is more specific than that and that it includes descriptors such as large breasts, long legs, and long hair. Regardless of the precise description, the body size associated with the thin ideal is significantly smaller than most women, which means that in order to achieve this ideal most women are told they would have to engage in some sort of intense and prolonged exercise and/or diet regime. Typically, however, such regimes are unsustainable and when discontinued results in regaining the weight that was lost along with additional pounds. Thus, she weighs more than she did prior to starting her diet or exercise program. Many individuals become dissatisfied with the weight gain and try another program only to experience weight loss and regain all over again. This process is commonly referred to as yo-yo dieting or weight cycling and can have significantly negative effects on the body as will be discussed later in this book.

The body type currently prized for males, the muscular ideal, is typically described as being lean and muscular. The idea is that muscles should be well developed and clearly visible due to low body fat. Although this body type itself is visually distinct from the thin ideal, the degree to which achieving this body is realistic is not much different than it is for females. Males' bodies are different from one another with respect to how easily they can build muscle and lose body fat. Thus, the predominant depiction of male bodies sporting the muscular ideal in magazines and other forms of media represents a standard that is far removed from what most males can achieve in a healthy manner. The results are similar to that of females: some males will engage in strict diet and exercise routines in order to achieve this look only to find that it is unsustainable. They will regain body fat that was lost and lose muscle mass—then repeat the process with another approach to try to achieve the allusive ideal.

What seems to be a strong predictor of whether or not males or females will engage in behaviors in pursuit of either ideal is something called internalization. Internalization refers to the process of buying into a concept or making that concept your own. For example, if you have the same beliefs about the world (whether political, religious, or otherwise) as your parents because they taught you these beliefs you have internalized them. Since the thin and muscular ideals predominate much of our culture, and friends and family members may think pursuing these standards is a good idea, it is not that unusual for us to internalize this ideal, make it our own, and pursue it in whatever way we are told will be effective. Many of us may even pursue the ideal regardless of health or well-being. It is not uncommon, for example, for women trying to become thinner to say that they would rather be skinny than healthy.

Internalization of the thin ideal or muscular ideal have each been identified as a risk factor for problems with body image and eating behaviors including those associated with eating disorders. Thus, the more strongly one believes the ideal should be achieved, the greater their risk for psychological problems.

IMPACT OF THE BODY SHAPE AND SIZE THAT IS CURRENTLY PRIZED

Just like any body ideal, the current ideal for male and female bodies puts forth a standard that not everyone can easily meet. As noted in the previous sections, some women of the 1900s had ribs removed so that they could attain the thin waist look of the day. Most people cannot meet the current ideals without engaging in some extreme behavior such as excessive weight loss and/or loss of body fat, excessive exercise whether aerobic or anaerobic, abuse of laxatives or diuretics, abuse of over-the-counter or prescription weight loss medications, or a new and particularly alarming trend among those with diabetes which is to not use their insulin doses as prescribed in order to control their weight. Many people are desperate to look like what is portrayed in magazines and other forms of media that they are willing to do whatever it takes to achieve this look.

Most people attempting to live up to the ideal standard for their sex will experience a significant hit to their self-esteem. Since we are told that achieving a particular look is something we should strive for, the further removed we are from that ideal the worse, we may feel about ourselves. Researchers poignantly illustrated this effect when they had female participants look at fashion magazines for 2–3 minutes. Participants' level of self-esteem was measured before and after looking at the magazines. The results showed that just a few minutes of looking through magazines showing the thin idea resulted in a measurable drop in self-esteem. This makes one wonder what the impact is on self-esteem over hours, days, and years of seeing these images and hearing about products and services you can buy to help you achieve the ideal? How serious can this pressure get? For a certain percentage of people, both male and female, this pressure can lead to significant mental health issues. One class of disorders that is highly associated with a focus on body shape and size is eating disorders. Since eating disorders have the highest mortality rate of any mental illness, this category of disorders is as serious as it gets. The decrease in body size among models in the 1980s and 1990s compared to previous decades has been found to correspond to a rise in incidence of eating disorders, which include anorexia nervosa, bulimia nervosa, and binge eating disorder (BED).

Anorexia nervosa involves someone losing a lot of weight to the point that they will eventually become significantly underweight. Bulimia nervosa is associated with the binge–purge cycle. This means that someone will eat a large quantity of food in a short amount of time then engage in a behavior (e.g., self-induced vomiting, excessive exercise, fasting) designed to get rid of the calories they ate. BED involves binging just like with bulimia nervosa but without engaging in any behavior to get rid of the calories. BED is believed to be the most commonly occurring eating disorder among the three and anorexia nervosa leads to significantly more deaths than the other two disorders.

Although eating disorders are usually associated with females, the reality is that more and more males are being diagnosed with eating disorders. There is no way yet to reliably predict who will develop an eating disorder and who will not; however, dieting puts people at much greater risk compared to those who do not diet. Those who diet for the purpose of trying to change their body weight and shape are also probably highly invested in the importance of the thin ideal or muscular ideal, which puts them at even greater risk for developing an eating disorder. Additionally, a disorder more commonly found among males seems to be on the rise and is strongly associated with the pursuit of the muscular ideal. It is a form of body dysmorphic disorder and is sometimes referred to as muscle dysmorphia or bigorexia. This disorder involves someone being so focused on muscle development that they will devote all available time and energy to the pursuit of "perfect" muscles. They will constantly scrutinize their bodies looking for imperfections and often see an imperfection that does not exist. They will then devote even more resources to "fixing" their body that they may start to skip school or work and let their relationships dissolve. Although muscle dysmorphia is not an eating disorder, it is often discussed in the context of eating disorder since there are similarities with respect to the investment of a particular ideal and a lot of effort directed to trying to change one's body shape and size.

Developing an eating disorder can have a profound impact on one's mental health and physical health. It is not uncommon for those with eating disorders to also be contending with other diagnosable psychiatric disorders. For example, anorexia nervosa is often diagnosed along with obsessive-compulsive disorder, and individuals diagnosed with bulimia nervosa may also have a co-occurring a substance use disorder. Although suicide in and of itself is not a formal diagnosis, suicidal thinking and suicidal attempts can coincide with eating disorders. In fact, among those with anorexia nervosa, suicide and heart failure are the two leading causes of death. In addition to the possibility of death as a result of an eating disorder, individuals often experience significant problems with their gastrointestinal system, which can be exacerbated with the abuse of laxatives. Malnutrition, either as a result of a starvation-based diet or severely limited variety of food, can lead to problems with skin, hair, nails, and bones. Osteoporosis or its precursor, osteopenia, can develop in those with anorexia nervosa regardless of age.

For those who do not develop a diagnosable eating disorder, there is a high probability that they will engage in a pattern of dieting for weight loss, regain the weight plus additional pounds, diet again, regain the weight plus additional pounds, diet again, and so on. As has been previously noted, this pattern is referred to as yo-yo dieting and is associated with significant health consequences such as being at increased risk for diabetes or heart disease.

As stated earlier, it is rare for most people to be able to achieve either ideal easily. This means that for almost all of us our natural body shape and size will not look the ideal. Trying to force our body to look like the ideal is not unlike trying to fit a square peg into a round hole. You can force the peg into the hole but since it is not designed to fit, the only way to make it fit is to exert a lot of pressure. If you are successful in making it fit, you probably did some damage in the process—some of which may not be reversible.

CHAPTER 2

Health and Body Mass Index (BMI)

An individual's body mass index (BMI) is often conflated with one's health. The thinking here is that if you, or anyone including a health-care professional, know your BMI then you also know how healthy you are. The subsequent assumption is that higher the BMI the less healthy someone is, and the lower the BMI the more healthy they are. A growing body of literature and anecdotal information has challenged this assumption.

This chapter will examine how health is defined as well as measured by leading health organizations. Readers will also learn what BMI actually is in terms of how it is calculated and why the measurement was developed in the first place (hint: it was not developed for the reasons it is used today in the medical field). In addition, BMI will be discussed in terms of costs associated with it and whether or not we have control over what BMI our bodies are. The remainder of the chapter will be devoted to the use of BMI in medical practices and how it is used to make decisions related to insurance. The chapter will conclude with a look at the fact that healthy and unhealthy individuals can be found at nearly all BMIs.

DEFINITION AND MEASUREMENT OF HEALTH

Those whose job it is to determine what resources are needed to help bolster a society's overall health must make a determination about the current health status of a society, and, based on demographic trends, make predictions about the overall health of the society in the future. For example, in the United States, as individuals are living longer and since the baby boomer generation is in its older adulthood years, it is likely that the prevalence of certain diseases will increase such as Alzheimer's dementia. This disease is projected to be more than twice as prevalent by the year 2030 as it was in 2006. The cost of caring for those with this disease will be felt not just by friends, family, and direct caregivers, but also by the society at large. Therefore, when a trend like this is projected, funds are directed to efforts designed to treat and prevent such diseases. Since there is an identifiable trend associated with weight in the United States, any impact weight may have on health becomes an important area of focus.

Definition of Health

The World Health Organization (WHO) defines health as "a state of complete physical, mental and social well-being and not merely the absence of disease or infirmity." Their website notes that this definition has not changed since 1948. The WHO's definition is one that is embraced by local governments as well as countries worldwide. The importance of this definition cannot be overstated since it is clear that a healthy person is not merely someone who isn't sick but someone who also has a high quality of life. Often times, however, when the health of a nation is discussed, it is often done so using the metrics of mortality or disease.

When health is defined by the rate of death within a population then the measurement of this aspect of health is to determine how many people die during a particular period of time. Mortality can be tracked by leading causes of death overall, by age, sex, or race, and so on. Another way to measure health is by assessing what is termed morbidity. Morbidity refers to the number of cases of particular disease in a population that do not lead to death. Currently, the only disease that cannot be spread via infection, on which the United States has this type of data, is cancer. Other ways that morbidity can be measured is via hospitalization rates for particular diseases and disorders, measurement of disability such as pain related to arthritis, chronic diseases such as heart and lung disease, mental health disorders, and disorders related to hearing and seeing. All of these methods, however, only speak about one part of the WHO's definition of health: the presence or absence of disease or infirmity. As the other portion of the WHO's definition indicates, another way to measure health is overall quality of life, which is noted to be particularly important when there are large numbers of disease processes that do not lead to death. Thus, people may be living longer but suffering a great deal, which would drastically lower their quality of life.

Measurement of Health

An article published in 2006 in the journal *Public Health Reports* indicates that regardless of how health is defined the measurement of it remains a tricky business. There is no one single measure of health that would encapsulate all elements of what it means to be healthy or unhealthy. The authors also note that the comparison of health-related data from one country to the next or one time period to the next can yield misleading results due to differences in how the data were measured and obtained. They also note that things such as procedures for being prepared for an emergency including a natural disaster or terrorist attack are typically not encapsulated in current measurements of health but would impact the overall health of a population should such an emergency occur. Moreover, the article states that while environmental quality, mental health, and socioeconomic status are generally regarded as impacting overall health, there do not exist precise metrics for assessing these factors and are therefore not often incorporated into public health programs. A recent effort involving multiple nations sought to standardize how health is conceptualized and measured, and how those results are communicated with others.

In June 2015, leaders from across the globe convened a Summit on the Measurement and Accountability for Results in Health in Washington, D.C. At this summit, The Roadmap for Health Measurement and Accountability was launched. The purpose of the roadmap was to identify the best strategies for assessing health programs in any country. This document not only looked at what health markers were important to measure but among them which ones should be focused on to best assess the health of a particular country. The authors of the roadmap recognized that the various countries would be more or less advanced with respect to their focus on health and their ability to effectively assess it. They noted, for example, that while many countries may exist in a digital age providing them easier access to a variety of types of data, other countries rely on paper systems and are far removed from being able to digitize the data they do have. A push to standardize a universal approach to the measurement of health would allow for more effective comparisons between countries as well as comparisons using data collected within a particular country from one year to the next. The architects of this roadmap identified seven strategic actions that were proposed as requirements of countries who intended to collect and report on health-related data. The seven strategic actions are as follows:

- Invest in strengthening data sources and capacities
- Align stakeholders in support of country health information systems

- Use the digital revolution to scale-up health interventions and engage civil society
- Strengthen public goods for health information and accountability
- Use data throughout all levels to improve policy, systems, and delivery
- Capture data on determinants of health as part of the country health information system
- Strengthen accountability and reporting of results

Overall the roadmap was developed to encourage those invested in the overall health and well-being of a particular population to direct resources toward effective measurement of health, to make sure all stakeholders are working toward the same goals, to make sure solid systems are in place making the collection health-related data a matter of routine, and to move data collection and storage to digital format for ease of use in analyzing and sharing data.

It is important to note that prior to this effort to standardize data collection and transmission of health-related data the United States recognized that electronically storing and transmitting data could put a patient's health-related information at risk of being tampered with or stolen. In 1996 the United States enacted the Health Insurance Portability and Accountability Act (HIPAA), which regulates, in part, how private health information is stored and shared. Those who have been to a health-care provider's office in the United States in recent years have signed a privacy form, which states how that office keeps private health information protected and private even when shared digitally (e.g., e-mail, fax). This form reflects how that particular office adheres to HIPAA. Any entity storing, using, or transmitting a patient's health-related information has to comply with HIPAA and inform consumers of how they will ensure that a patient's health information will be kept private.

Regardless of the precise definition of health used by any nation, or the manner in which health-related data might be collected, one particular demographic variable has the attention of policy makers, schools, and health-care professionals. The steady increase in weight among citizens of the United States and other countries, along with particular disease processes associated with larger body sizes, has thrust a concept known as BMI into the health spotlight.

ORIGIN AND DEFINITION OF BMI

BMI stands for *body mass index* and is the current metric used by many health-care professionals to determine the degree of one's health. BMI is relatively easy to calculate and was originally developed using the metric system. The formula is:

$$\frac{\text{Weight in kilograms}}{\text{Height in meters}^2}$$

$$\frac{\text{Weight in pounds} \times 703}{\text{Height in inches}^2}$$

BMI has been strongly linked to a variety of disease processes such as diabetes, hypertension, and heart disease. Since BMI is easy enough to compute with a calculator but even more expedient if a computer is used, it is no wonder BMI is relied upon by most health-care providers as a quick and easy way to capture one's overall health. Height and weight are easily measured and are therefore difficult to manipulate. When weight manipulation does occur, for example, it is often in the context of anorexia nervosa and the individual may try to appear heavier than they actually are in order to avoid having to eat or undergo a more intensive form of treatment (e.g., inpatient or residential). Despite the widespread use of BMI to determine an *individual's* degree of health, the origins of BMI indicate it was developed for a different purpose.

BMI was developed in 1832 and was originally referred to as the Quetelet Index after its developer Adolphe Quetelet who was reportedly on a quest to measure the "average man." Dr. Quetelet, a Belgian, earned his doctorate at the age of 23 in mathematics and developed an interest in probabilities. He applied this area of inquiry to understanding various characteristics of human beings including physical characteristics like the relationship between height and weight. He later extended the application of his theories to understanding human behavior. His interest in collecting and calculating statistical data lead him to organize the first International Statistical Congress in 1853. A result of this effort was the development of the precursor to what is now known as the International Classification of Diseases (ICD) used in the medical field. The ICD is used internationally, including the United States, to identify particular medical and psychiatric diseases. As of 2016 the ICD is in its 10th edition and is scheduled to be published in its 11th edition in 2018.

In his pursuit of trying to understand and quantify human characteristics, Dr. Quetelet developed the Quetelet Index, but his overall interest was in understanding the relationship between height and weight in the human population as a whole not in individual human beings. Additionally, despite the index's current use, Dr. Quetelet was not interested in obesity. His focus was on determining what was most representative of a normal person and couching that within a distribution of measurements that were not normal. The Quetelet Index retained this moniker until 1972 when Ancel Keys renamed it the body mass index and ultimately became the method for determining someone's obesity status.

Ancel Keys devoted much of his career to studying and understanding how body mass affected the health and well-being of the human body. One of his most well-known studies, published in the mid-1940s, was entitled "Human Starvation and Its Consequences," and is often cited by researchers and clinicians when discussing the effects of reduced caloric intake. The Human Starvation study was conducted in large part to understand the effects of those confined to the concentration camps of World War II. Dr. Keys' findings are still cited in articles on the study of anorexia nervosa and other eating disorders involving severely reduced caloric intake and dramatic weight loss.

In 1972 Keys published an article entitled "Indices of Relative Weight and Obesity" in which he argued that the formula widely used at the time to understand the weight to height ratio was inadequate. At the time, a formula called the *ponderal index* was used and it is as follows:

$$\frac{\text{Weight (kg)}}{\text{height (m)}^3}$$

Keys argued that this formula did not take into consideration the fact that the human body would not necessarily look the same from one height to the next. He asserted that the Quetelet Index would more accurately quantify the relationship between weight and height in human beings. It was at this time Keys renamed the Quetelet Index as the body mass index.

BMI is widely used today; however, in recent years it has come under fire as being a poor indicator of the health of any single person. Those who argue against the use of BMI as a measure of one's health remind us that in his quest to understand the average man Adolphe Quetelet developed his formula in an effort to study and understand populations. He never intended his index to be applied to individuals. Additionally, a recent study conducted out of UCLA examined health-related data collected between the years 2005 and 2012 on over 40,000 people. They looked at BMI and test results that would indicate problems related to heart disease, diabetes, and overall inflammation. The researchers found that just over 47 percent of those with a BMI in the overweight range and almost 30 percent of those classified as obese were metabolically healthy. Equally important was their finding that over 30 percent of those categorized as having a normal BMI showed indicators that they were not metabolically healthy. This is one study among many have been accumulating over recent years calling into question the use of BMI as a reflection of one's overall health. Despite such evidence, BMI continues to play a prominent role in the medical records of most people in the United States.

USES OF BMI IN MEDICINE

Growth Charts and Medical Records

Growth charts are used by medical providers to track the physical development of children from birth to age 20 to determine if they are growing at an expected and healthy rate. Currently, growth charts are different for boys and girls, and therefore the growth curve (i.e., the line one gets when connecting data points on a graph) is expected to be different between the sexes. The focus of this section is on the growth charts that are related to height and weight; however, there are also growth charts for plotting the growth of head circumference for children from birth to 24 months. The growth charts in use today for measuring weight and height have changed substantially from those that were used in the past. Visually they may appear to be similar; however, the data used to indicate what healthy growth looks like when plotted on a graph is quite disparate.

Growth charts of one variety or another have been used in the United States since the early 1900s; however, the data used to establish what was considered normal or healthy growth were not representative of age, ethnicity, socioeconomic status, variations in genetics, the environment, or geography that many citizens of the United States could be exposed to. Thus, the charts were useful only in understanding the growth of a very narrow subset of the population. For example, the charts used for 30 years from the mid-1940s to the mid-1970s, known as the *Stuart/Meredith Growth Charts,* were based on a sample of non-Hispanic white children who lived near Iowa City, Iowa, or Boston, Massachusetts.

In the early to mid-1970s, various professional groups including the American Academy of Pediatrics, the Maternal and Child Health Program of the Bureau of Community Health Services, and the U.S. Public Health Service noted the need for new growth charts that would more accurately represent the entire population of the United States. When these new charts were developed by the National Center for Health Statistics (NCHS), they were based on data collected from different sources but that were also far more representative of the national population. Thus, in 1977 NCHS produced 14 charts based on age (birth up to age 18) and sex. These charts are generally referred to as the *1977 NCHS Growth Charts*. In 1978, the Centers for Disease Control and Prevention (CDC) used a statistical procedure to normalize the expected growth curve for these charts which allowed users of the charts to determine more accurately what was average for a given age and sex and what constituted measurements that were significantly different than the average. These normalized charts were ultimately recommended for international use by the WHO.

Critics of the 1977 charts and 1978 normalized charts pointed out that at least one study used to develop the charts was still conducted on a demographically narrow subset of the population (i.e., formula-fed, white, middle-class infants living in one area of Ohio). They also indicated that this study measured infant growth at intervals that could miss important developmental changes. Data were collected at birth and one month, at three-month intervals from 3 to 12 months of age, and at six-month intervals from 12 to 36 months of age. Since a child's development rapidly changes in the first several years of life, it was argued that the lengthy intervals in between data collection could not adequately capture normal development. Other criticisms of 1977/1978 growth charts included the fact that growth beyond age 18 could not be tracked on these charts, which was considered to be problematic since many people continue to physically develop into their 20s. Finally, these growth charts did not allow for measurements at the extremes of height and weight (i.e., measurements beyond the 5th and 95th percentiles). Therefore, a call for revised charts was once again issued based on the fact that more current and comprehensive data were available on the U.S. population, and more sophisticated statistical procedures had been developed which would more accurately determine a normal growth curve for individuals by age and sex.

In the year 2000, the CDC published a report recommending the adoption of new growth charts developed using more recently collected data and improved statistics. Improvements included a more demographically representative data set, the ability to track data up to the age of 20, and the ability to plot data ranging from the 3rd to 97th percentiles. These new charts, which are still in use today, included sex-specific infant charts for weight for age and recumbent length (i.e., lying down) for age. The child and adolescent charts are also sex-specific including measurements for weight by age and stature (i.e., standing up) by age. Thus, just like previous charts, the 2000 growth charts allow medical providers and parents to see how a child's growth progresses from year to year, and also how their weight and height (or length) growth compares to other children of the same sex and age. These growth charts were also the first to include BMI as a measurement.

BMI was included on the new growth charts to help professionals identify children who could be at risk for being overweight or obese as they aged. Currently, a child or teenager is considered overweight if their weight measures at the 85th percentile or less than the 95th percentile based on age and sex, and they are considered obese if at or above the 95th percentile. Although fully grown adults no longer require the use of growth charts, the CDC recommends that BMI is calculated and recorded by their primary care provider (PCP). Overweight and obesity for adults is not based on percentages but rather on the BMI measurement itself. An adult, regardless of sex, with a BMI of 25.0 to 29.9 is considered over-weight and an adult with a BMI of 30.0 or higher is considered obese. These standards, however, have not always been set where they are today. From 1985 to 1998, the cutoff for BMI criteria indicating an adult was overweight was 27.8 for men and 27.3 for women. When the BMI cut-off for overweight was lowered from 27 to 25 in June 1998 people took notice. Many people observed what CNN noted: "Millions of Americans became 'fat' Wednesday—even if they didn't gain a pound." Tens of mil-lions Americans who were identified as normal weight or healthy one day literally became overweight or unhealthy overnight. The *American Jour-nal of Clinical Nutrition* noted that when this change in criteria was made the number of overweight adults went from 61.7 million to 97.1 million—an increase of 35.4 million adults highlighting the dramatic effect a change in cutoff can have.

Based on their classification of overweight or obese, medical providers often recommend weight loss to improve one's health given the numer-ous studies that have linked heavier weight with various ailments from joint pain to heart disease and the assumption that body size is an effective proxy for health. Thus, the reclassification of BMI cutoffs for overweight and obesity had significant implications not only for diagnosis but also for treatment. Since the recommendation is almost always weight loss for someone identified as overweight or obese, assistance for helping peo-ple lose weight can include medication (whether prescribed by one's PCP or purchased over-the-counter), increase in exercise, decrease in caloric intake, decrease in consumption of certain types of foods, weight-loss sur-gery designed limit the body's ability to metabolize food, or some com-bination of these methods. These are big businesses with the amount of money spent on weight loss related products and procedures estimated at over $60 billion a year.

BMI AND HEALTH INSURANCE COMPANIES

Health insurance companies are businesses. While they provide a ser-vice it is a paid service and most companies are invested in maximizing income while minimizing payouts. It is, therefore, in the best interests of an insurance company to identify who may be at greater risk of using their health-care benefits as a result of existing conditions, medical risk for developing future conditions, and those who may engage in high-risk behaviors thereby jeopardizing their health. Overweight and obesity are criteria used to establish risk in a particular individual.

Costs associated with higher BMIs

Obesity has long been identified as a costly condition. An article published in *Obesity Research* in 1998 reported that the overall cost of obesity in the United States was believed to be just over $99 billion and about $51 billion was attributed to cost related to medical care. In 1997 Canadians, by contrast, reported that costs that were the direct result of obesity was just under $2 billion (Canadian dollars). While publications like this would appear to indicate that weight loss itself will lower the costs of being obese, other studies paint a different picture. One study of BMI, physical activity, and the cost of health-care among retirees in the United States found that if retirees were physically active they would pay less than their less active counterparts including those in the normal weight range. Despite studies like this indicating that it might be physical activity or the lack thereof that contributes to the use of health-care, obesity is pointed to as the reason health-care costs are so high. That cost is often passed along to individuals seeking insurance regardless of whether or not medical tests indicate they are healthy. Many obese individuals are penalized for having a BMI that is too high resulting in these individuals paying more for insurance than someone who is similar to them in other ways but who has a lower BMI.

Most people purchase health insurance to take care of themselves and their family should a major medical issue arise. The reality is that insurance companies are businesses that are interested in not only making money but being sure that those who are at greater risk of using their health-care policies pay more for the privilege of having insurance coverage. Thus, insurance companies are very interested in data and statistics that indicate who is at greater risk of developing problems that would require the use of their insurance. Having this data readily available allows companies to easily determine if a potential customer is someone who is risky for them to take on and, if so, they will pay more to have insurance coverage. Similarly, if someone engages in high-risk behaviors such as sky diving or rock climbing then they can expect to pay more along with those who are regular smokers. These behaviors, of course, are self-reported and can be falsified. Certainly if one experiences major injury as a result of jumping out of an airplane and the insurance company was not informed the insurance company will probably not pay for the medical costs. One's weight and height and ultimately BMI, however, are easily measured by a medical professional who can then provide this information to the insurance company. This is one reason why weight or BMI is so often used as a risk factor—it is easily and objectively measured.

In 1994 a researcher out of England reported that due to the connection of obesity to various medical issues including coronary heart disease and overall shorter life-span obesity is believed to cause an increase in what is spent on health-care, a decrease in lifespan, a decrease in work-related productivity, and retiring earlier than would be expected. This researcher further concluded that health insurance companies should take this into consideration when developing insurance policies. Recent research, however, has begun to challenge some of these claims. For example, studies have suggested that a BMI in the normal range is not necessarily as protective as previously thought. For example, a recent study conducted in 2015 by D. H. Chenoweth found that those with a BMI between 23 and 29 (that's the upper end of normal and the entire range for overweight) are less likely to die prematurely than those with other BMIs. Another study found that medical care costs may be lowest for those with BMIs between 25 and 27 (which is in the overweight classification). Another recent study found that a significant percentage of normal weight individuals were metabolically unhealthy and an even larger percentage of those overweight or obese were found to be metabolically healthy. These studies and others provide evidence that BMI itself is not likely the best indicator of one's current or future health and may also indicate that those with too high a BMI may be inappropriately identified as risky customers. One insurance company published an article entitled *How Does BMI Affect Life Insurance Rates?* This company noted that a high BMI found in highly trained athletes is probably a false positive for someone who is a risky customer since muscle mass weighs more than fat. They noted that someone with a high muscle ratio resulting in a high BMI could have their rates adjusted so they are not overpaying providing that other health indicators "are in line with preferred rate requirements." Meaning that as long as all other indicators of a healthy body are present a high BMI will not penalize those with a high muscle ratio. No such exception was offered for those with a high BMI who do not have a high muscle ratio but can demonstrate that all other health indicators "are in line with preferred rate requirements." A recent study demonstrates that this is quite possible.

A study in 2015 was conducted to look at whether or not BMI is at all related to how much worker's compensation was used. They concluded

that higher BMIs were connected to more lost workdays and higher indem-
nity costs (i.e., how much the insurance has to pay to the employee) and
indicated that employers implement programs that target obesity in their
employees. What this did not account for, however, were other factors that
may have contributed to these findings. For example, recent research has
begun to find that being sedentary throughout the day on most days may
be far more hazardous to one's health than having a larger body. Thus, it
is possible that the true cause of the increase in workers' compensation
claims was not body size but being too sedentary on the job. The authors
noted that they did not specifically look at the degree to which someone's
job is sedentary, which they also noted could have had an impact on claims.

Despite newer research casting doubt on the declaration that being
obese is costly fiscally as well as physically, many continue to point to the
extensive literature suggesting that higher BMIs are indeed more costly
and that these costs are a burden to society at large. When relying on this
data for decision making, an important factor to consider is whether or not
the research proves cause and effect or whether or not the research simply shows that two or more factors are connected in some way. The latter
is referred to as correlational research and only reveals a connection or
relationship between factors but not which one may have caused the other
one. This is an important point because when decisions are made about
who should be financially penalized because they are a greater burden
on society it is important to know that the correct cause of that burden is
identified. The kicker with correlational research is that it is not possible
to determine what the cause is. When BMI is associated with a higher cost
to insurance or society at large the assumption made by most people is that
BMI itself is the cause of the increased burden. The reality is that the current research does not reveal this. There are many factors that contribute
to someone's height and weight, not the least of which is genetics, but also
lifestyle. There are also many factors that contribute to diseases that have
been associated with higher BMIs like diabetes and heart disease. When
we find that there is a relationship between two things and then decide that
one of those things is the cause for the other, we are not only misrepresent-
ing the data and the science but also probably missing a significant piece
(or pieces) of what is actually causing particular disease processes.

To illustrate the importance of knowing what is really going on with
two pieces of information we can look at correlations that are quite strong
but would be ridiculous to conclude that one factor is the cause of the
other. A perfect correlation is 1.00. This means that every single time one
thing occurs, the other thing also occurs. So the closer a correlation is to

1.00 the stronger the relationship. Here are some examples of very strong correlations, but that most people would not mistakenly think of in terms of cause and effect:

- Revenue generated by arcades and the number of doctoral degrees in computer science in the United States has a correlation of .98. This means that the more revenue arcades produce the more doctorates in computer science there are in the United States. This is one of these studies that could easily generate a media title of something like "Want a Ph.D. in computer science? Spend a lot of money on arcade games."
- Another correlation that reached a near perfect relationship at .99 was found between the divorce rate in Maine and the amount of margarine that was consumed per capita. "Live in Maine and don't want a divorce? Don't eat margarine." Or, of course, "Live in Maine and looking to get out of your marriage? Eat a lot of margarine."

These headlines, hopefully, sound ridiculous. Hopefully readers would think it is ridiculous to conclude that eating more margarine would *cause* someone to get a divorce, or that spending a lot of money on arcade games would *cause* someone to earn a Ph.D. in computer science, but that is precisely what these fictitious headlines imply. They suggest a cause-and-effect relationship where there is none. It becomes trickier to convince people that a strong relationship between two things does not mean that one causes the other one if it confirms what they already think or if it is just common sense. This seems to be the case with obesity. Since most people believe that being overweight or obese causes a greater financial burden on society or causes one to develop various diseases sensationalized headlines based on correlational research such as "Being overweight linked to poorer memory" or "Bariatric surgery associated with reduction in cardiovascular events and death" fuel these beliefs.

This is, unfortunately, what is happening with many of the studies conducted on BMI. There is no doubt that strong relationships (i.e., correlations) exist between BMI and a multitude of other things like various diseases and even costs associated with health care. The problem exists when this data is used to make the case that higher BMIs are the cause of the diseases or the rise in health-care costs. What if it isn't? Perhaps it really is the cause of these things, but as of the writing of this book, data supporting these claims in the form of studies examining cause and effect do not exist.

Additional Factors Related to Insurance Coverage

In addition to higher premium costs for those with a BMI deemed too high, those who do have insurance and who may engage in weight loss efforts may not have those efforts covered by their insurance. For example, the costly group of weight loss surgeries known as bariatric surgery may not be covered by all insurances. The issue of the role insurance companies may play when it comes to weight related recommendations dates back more than 60 years.

In 1952, Hope Grosse wrote an article in which she noted that the two most common reasons an insurance policy would be loaded (i.e., how much is built into the cost of the insurance) were weight and/or blood pressure that was above average, and age. She goes on to state that it is not clear where the line is with respect to when a blood pressure or weight is too high; however, she suggests that the medical officer evaluating someone for insurance purposes would rely on their clinical expertise but that ultimately the insurance underwriter (i.e., not a medical professional) would make the final determination regarding how much a particular insurance policy should cost.

In this article, she acknowledges that two individuals of the same age and height who eat the same amount and type of food might wind up with different body sizes. But, nonetheless recommends that the larger person must realize his "handicap" and "grin and bear it" by severely restricting what they eat. She also notes that there is such a thing as a "normal weight" and that to maintain it one must eat the right amount of food implying that if someone winds up with a larger body they are clearly eating too much and need to cut back. She further notes that weight reduction remains an important part of treatment for those identified as obese. Despite saying that the purpose of the article is not to explicate *how* to lose weight she goes on to talk about what effect eliminating potatoes, bread, or butter may have on weight.

Not much has changed in over 60 years since this article was written. Weight loss is still an often recommended treatment for those who are obese, regardless of what may have brought them to see their physician or contributed to their body being large. Moreover, recommendations about how to lose weight often espouse the "calories in, calories out" mantra, while also recommending that certain foods be eliminated completely or at least highly restricted in one's food intake. The notion of what people are or are not doing with regards to their health has direct bearing on health insurance coverage. Of course what is not agreed upon is which behaviors constitute unhealthy behaviors.

One area of interest when it comes to health insurance is a concept known as *moral hazard*. Moral hazard refers to how someone behaves if they are protected from experiencing harm. In other words, if someone is covered by health insurance will they keep doing what they've always been doing or will they engage in more risky behavior since if something bad does happen they are covered? In 2009 researchers Kelly and Markowitz examined this very question with respect to obesity. They wanted to know if people, when covered by health insurance, would engage in behaviors that would increase their chances of gaining weight. The results of their study indicated that people were more likely to be classified as overweight, but not obese, if they were covered by health insurance. They acknowledged that their finding reflected a small effect and the average weight gain among those studied was 1.8 pounds. Thus, if you are covered by health insurance you are likely to be nearly 2 pounds heavier than if you did not have health insurance. Although this finding was statistically significant which in the world of research means that the effect is not due to chance, it is debatable whether or not the finding is meaningful. Nonetheless, it is a finding that can be used to influence who is covered and how much it costs especially if the summary of the article is: people will engage in behaviors that contribute to being heavier if they have health insurance. The researchers concluded, however, that although behaviors affecting one's health seem to be connected to health insurance one is not necessarily a cause of the other. This is an important statement as it acknowledges the fact that even though two things might be found to be connected (e.g., when people have insurance their behaviors change) it does not mean that one has *caused* the other one to happen.

WHAT CONTROL DO WE HAVE OVER CHANGING OUR BMI?

"Calories in-calories out." That is the mantra repeated by many who are in the midst of a diet or exercise plan. It is the rationale provided by many health-care professionals for why weight loss is relatively simple and straightforward. All you have to do is eat less than the energy you expend or exercise more than the calories you eat (of course the reverse is true for gaining weight) and you will lose weight. Diets of any variety capitalize on the calories in/calories out notion since most diets encourage calorie restriction. Thus, even if you do not increase your exercise you should lose weight because you are eating less. It then becomes tempting to think that if eating "this amount" resulted in "this amount" of weight lost, then eating even fewer calories will result in even more weight lost. In the short term this appears to be true enough. There are a number of problems with this approach, however, not the least of which includes the question: At what point do you or should you stop losing weight?

Another factor that is often overlooked in our pursuit of weight loss is a concept known as weight set point. One's weight set point refers to the weight your particular body should be given your age, sex, and height. This is the weight at which your body will settle when you fuel it properly (i.e., consume a variety of foods in sufficient quantities) and engage in regular physical activity. Not everyone's set point will be the same, however, when engaging in the same eating and exercise behaviors. Some of us will be heavier than others and some will be lighter than others—regardless of age, sex, and height. This translates to a significant percentage of the population that is far removed objectively and aesthetically from the thin or muscular ideal.

There are a multitude of factors that contribute to whether or not any of us are able to lose weight and keep it off in the long term. There are structures in our brain, for example, that control our feelings of satiety. These brain structures initiate processes that result in physiological signals we have learned to interpret as "I'm hungry" or "I'm full." It can, therefore, feel as if we can control what and how much we eat from meal to meal. We simply need to exert this control or willpower and we will be successful. These same mechanisms, however, are also working overtime not just from one meal to the next but over longer periods of time. This helps to explain why many people can eliminate or severely restrict certain types of food or restrict overall calorie amounts for a finite amount of time before they experience cravings that cause them to cheat or fail. We interpret giving in to these cravings as personal failures when in reality the brain has been monitoring things for quite some time and has determined that intake has been insufficient. The body will then send out stronger signals than normal telling us that not only does eating need to occur now, but eating needs to include foods that will help the person gain weight. Historically, after periods of famine human beings have feasted on as much food as possible in order to store up fat as an energy source for when famine hits again. These mechanisms are still in place even if the famine is self-imposed through dieting.

Another factor affecting weight loss is one's metabolism. Roughly speaking, one's metabolism refers to the rate at which the body uses energy. The basal metabolic rate refers to how much energy your body uses when you are at rest. The more your body uses the more efficient your metabolism, the less your body uses the less efficient your metabolism.

Our individual metabolisms, however, are not immovable. It is not the case that if you have an efficient metabolism you will always have an efficient metabolism. What your metabolism is to start with is largely determined by genetics; however, age will impact this and over time your metabolism will slow. Engaging in regular exercise can also affect the efficiency with which your body uses food usually resulting in a more efficient metabolism. How much one eats also affects your metabolism.

The body is wired to survive. It wants to live. Thus, when you restrict how much you eat, such as through dieting, to the point that you are consuming less than what your body uses in a day and you do this for a prolonged period of time eventually your body will recognize that there is not enough food and therefore will hang on to whatever food it can by slowing down your metabolism (i.e., burning fewer calories). Increasing intake again can result in an increase in metabolism (i.e., burning more calories). Related to this is a pattern of weight loss and weight gain that is often referred to as yo-yo dieting or weight cycling. Engaging in a pattern of weight loss and weight gain means that your metabolism is cycling through speeding up and slowing down. Over a long period of time, changes in metabolism can be permanent and usually result in a slower rather than a more efficient metabolism. Additionally, yo-yo dieting has negative health consequences associated with it. Those who have a history of yo-yo dieting may be at greater risk for developing diabetes, heart disease, and some forms of cancer.

Stress is another factor associated with weight gain that many readers may be familiar with. When under stress, stress hormones (e.g., cortisol, epinephrine) are released in large part to get your body prepared for the fight or flight response which is a response of the sympathetic nervous system that prepares the body to take action when there is danger. Although most sources of stress in the United States do not constitute actual danger (i.e., your life is not threatened), the brain does not know the difference and responds to all indications of danger in the same way. The long and short of it is that the release of stress hormones results in fat storage if the energy released by these hormones goes unused—which is usually the case with daily stress. Thus, the more stress you experience the greater the chance that you will experience weight gain.

Additional factors that affect weight include amount and quality of sleep, bacteria that exist in our digestive system, and even certain viruses. Thus, manipulating one's weight is not nearly as simple as calories in/calories out, and our incessant pursuit of the perfect diet may lead to yo-yo dieting which can backfire and ultimately cause weight gain not to mention may put our physical well-being at risk.

The Normal (Bell) Curve and How It Applies to BMI

The normal curve or bell curve is a specific graphic representation of data. Students of math and statistics may be familiar with the term and the appearance of this particular curve which resembles the shape of a bell. This curve represents what is called a *normal distribution,* which allows us to predict with a good deal of confidence where most data will be plotted. The normal curve is usually shown with several vertical lines dissecting the curve at various points. The line in the exact middle of the curve represents the mean or the statistical average of the data. On the normal curve 50 percent of the data fall on the right-hand side of the mean and 50 percent of the data fall on the left-hand side of the mean. Thus, the center line divides the data precisely in half.

There are three more lines on either side of the middle line and each line is the same distance from one another. Each line represents what is called the standard deviation which is a mathematical descriptor of how spread out the data are. It also provides an indication of how unusual a particular data point is (the further away from the middle a data point is, the more unusual it is). The lines on the right-hand side of the middle line represent positive (+) standard deviations, and the lines on the left-hand side represent negative (–) deviations. These lines also give us an indication of how much of the data falls between the lines. For example, approximately 68 percent of the data fall between the first lines on either side of the middle line (i.e., between –1 and +1 standard deviations) and 95 percent of the data fall between the second lines on either side of the middle line (i.e., between –2 and +2 standard deviations). We also know that only 2 percent of the data falls between the second and third lines on either side of the middle line (i.e., between –2 and –3 standard deviations *or* between +2 and +3 standard deviations).

Many measurable characteristics of human beings are believed to be accurately represented by the normal curve. Therefore, if we could gather data on all adults, for example, and plot the data on a graph we would find that around 68 percent of the population would cluster around the middle of the graph, and fewer and fewer members of the population would be represented on either extreme of the graph. BMI is believed, by some, to be represented by the normal curve. However, by others BMI is thought to be skewed.

A skewed distribution looks like when someone grabs the top of the bell curve (i.e., the highest point on the graph) and pulls it either to the right or to the left. A positively skewed graph has the top of the curve pulled to the left, which means that the statistical average is also pulled to the left. A negatively skewed graph has the top of the curve pulled to the right along with the statistical average.

As already noted, some researchers have presented BMI as a normal distribution meaning that regardless of what the average BMI is half of the population will fall to the right of, or will have a higher BMI than, average, and the other half of the population will fall to the left of, or will have a lower BMI than, average. Others have suggested that the distribution of BMI across the population is negatively skewed meaning that the statistical average would be pulled in the direction of a higher BMI. Researchers have suggested that the degree to which BMI is negatively skewed has increased over time. They account for this by pointing to what is known about how the body works with respect to weight gain and weight regulation: the heavier someone is already the easier it is for them to put on more weight. Thus, over time heavier people will gain more weight than lighter people resulting in a more strongly skewed distribution of weight and BMI.

Since the prevailing assumption is that those with higher BMIs will also have more significant health problems the shape of the distribution of BMI has direct implications for those who draft and implement public health policy, who provide direct care, and who study causes and effects of BMI. If we are growing larger (as measured by BMI) as a country over time and BMI is represented on a normal curve then that means that over time the entire curve is simply pushed to the right. The overall shape of the distribution doesn't change meaning that everyone is getting bigger at the same rate. If this is the trend, then the recommendation would be to apply prevention and treatment strategies to the entire population since every BMI would be increasing by the same amount. If, on the other hand, the distribution of BMI scores over time becomes more and more positively skewed that would mean that those with higher BMIs to start with would be gaining weight at a higher rate than those who started with lower BMIs. Practically speaking, that would suggest that prevention and intervention strategies ought to be applied only to those on the higher end of the distribution (i.e., those who started out with higher BMIs and whose BMIs would increase more rapidly). In many respects, this is what is happening since prevention and treatment efforts are targeted toward those who have a higher than normal BMI, meaning that they are already overweight or obese.

Another way in which the concept of the normal curve can be applied to BMI is with respect to looking at those classified as overweight or obese and plotting how unhealthy they are. The assumption has been that all or nearly all of those classified as obese would be unhealthy resulting in a heavily negatively skewed distribution of health among obese individuals. That is, far more people who are obese would be shown to have a lot of health problems and very few if any would be shown to be quite healthy. Recent research examining data collected on thousands of people suggest that the distribution of health may not be a skewed as has been assumed since just under 30 percent of obese individuals were found to be healthy rather than unhealthy.

CHAPTER 3

Rates of Obesity and Targeted Prevention Efforts

Overall rates of obesity have continued to climb over the past several years. Part of the explanation for that is the fact that our bodies are getting larger. Another part of that is changes made by the CDC to the BMI cutoff for overweight and obesity. When this change was made, over 34 million people who were previously considered to be normal weight were now in the overweight category. Increase in the overweight and obesity rates as a result of changes in criteria coupled with the increase in research showing that those who are obese may not be as unhealthy as previously though begs the question of whether or not the rise in obesity is truly something that deserves the label of epidemic and whether or not a war needs to be waged on body size. Before getting to those more controversial issues, the following sections examine how the rates of obesity are distributed among various demographics, what efforts have been made to address the rates of obesity, and what treatments are currently recommended to reduce obesity on a person-by-person basis.

This chapter will show how BMI is represented among various demographics including age, race, education level, and level of income. It will also examine how BMI is viewed socio-politically by taking a look at ad campaigns that target obesity, school policies that include BMI Report Cards, how BMI is invoked in politics, how public health-care policies are affected by concerns over the obesity rate especially among children, and how people with higher BMIs are discriminated against simply based on body size. The chapter will conclude with a look at what treatments the medical field provides for individuals who are overweight or obese, and how safe and effective these treatments are.

How Different Demographics Are Represented

Rates of obesity are not equal among different demographics. For example, despite the concern about childhood obesity adults have a higher rate of obesity than children and adolescents. Additionally, obesity rates are not equivalent between the sexes or among different racial groups, educational levels, or income levels.

Age

When considering obesity by age, the lowest rate is found among infants and children up to age two. The rates then climb steadily with age. Those who write about obesity statistics state that regardless of the relative stability of rates over the last 10–15 years the obesity rate is too high and that obesity rates should continue to be monitored and prevention efforts continued to be developed to bring the overall rate of obesity among U.S. citizens to much lower levels.

The highest incidence of obesity is among adults with about one-third of all adults in the United States identified as obese. The age group that has received the most attention, however, when it comes to the media, development of prevention strategies, and development of effective interventions, is children. The consensus among policy makers and medical providers is that obesity rates in children will lead to continued obesity in adulthood and an increase in obesity-related diseases at younger ages.

WHO growth charts are what the CDC recommends for use to determine what constitutes obesity for infants and children up to 2 years old. Children in this age range who are identified as measuring at or above the 95th percentile on the male or female growth chart based on their weight and recumbent length (i.e., how long they are when lying down) are classified as obese. At age 2 and above, use of CDC growth charts is recommended. Instead of recumbent length the child's or adolescent's standing height and weight are used to calculate BMI. Children aged 2 and above including adolescents up to age 19 are considered obese if their BMI is at or above the 95th percentile on the male or female growth charts. For adults (aged 20 years and older), obesity is simply identified based on actual BMI rather than whether or not one's BMI is equal to or higher than 95 percent of all other adults. Thus, obesity is identified in an adult when his or her BMI is at or above 30 (see Chapter 2 for how BMI is calculated).

The CDC reports trends in obesity going back to 1999–2000. At that time youth, ages 2–19, had an obesity rate of 13.9 percent and adults, ages 20+, had an obesity rate of 30.5 percent. Between then and the most recent data reported in 2013–2014, the obesity rates of youth and adults both increased to 17.2 percent and 37.7 percent, respectively. As of 2011–2012, infants and children up to age 2 had an obesity rate of just over 8 percent; children and adolescents ranging in age from 2 to 19 were reported as having an obesity rate of 17 percent, and adults were at a rate of 35 percent during the same time frame. These numbers represent rates that are essentially unchanged since 2003–2004. It is interesting to note, however, that children ages 2–5 years have shown a decrease in obesity rates from just under 14 percent in 2003–2004 to just under 8.5 percent in 2011–2012. During the later time frame children ages 6–11 years old had a much higher rate of obesity at over 17.5 percent and adolescents aged 12–19 had a rate of 20.5 percent. Thus, the overall rate of obesity of 17 percent for children seems to be primarily accounted for by children 6 years and older.

When looking at data from 2011 to 2014, the CDC reports that the obesity rates for adults has increased slightly to 36 percent, whereas the obesity rate for youth (ages 2–19) remained stable at 17 percent. Among adults there seems to be some differences in obesity rates during the 2011–2014 time frame. Middle-aged adults (40–59 years old) had an obesity rate of just over 40 percent and older adults aged 60 years and above had an obesity rate of 37 percent. Younger adults, aged 20–39 accounted for the lowest obesity rate at around 32 percent. The differences between middle-aged and older adults was statistically insignificant meaning the difference in rates is not meaningful and can be considered essentially the same rate; however, the rate of obesity among younger adults is considered to be significantly, or meaningfully different form the other two adult age ranges. Thus, it can be concluded that younger adults have an obesity rate that is lower than middle-aged and older adults.

As we'll see in the next few sections in this chapter, the overall numbers based on age paint one picture of obesity rates, but there are some differences based on sex, race and ethnicity, income level, and education level than may impact how prevention and intervention efforts are devised and implemented.

Sex

Public discussions of obesity often focus exclusively on obesity rates based on age and usually divide the population into two groups: children and adults. When looking more closely at the data there are additional differences within the various age ranges based on sex which may further impact how prevention and intervention strategies are developed and implemented.

As noted in the previous section, the overall obesity rate among adults in the years 2011–2014 was 36 percent and in youth the rate was 17 percent. Although there were no differences identified in rates of obesity between male and female youths, there was a difference between the sexes in adults. Adult women in this time frame had an obesity rate of just over 38 percent, whereas adult males had a rate of just over 34 percent. When examining the various stages of adulthood there are differences between the sexes; however, among children and adolescents the differences between males and females is much less dramatic.

For youth ages 2–19 years old, both males and females showed the lowest rage of obesity during the preschool years (ages 2–5). Boys had a rate of 9.2 percent and girls had a rate of 8.6 percent, which is a difference between the sexes that is not meaningful. Similarly, the differences between sexes were not meaningful at any other youth age range meaning that at all age categories among youth (i.e., 2–5 years, 6–11 years, and 12–19 years) there were no differences in obesity rates between males and females. However, obesity rates for both males and females in the 6–11 years (17.6% and 17.5%, respectively) and 12–19 years (20.1% and 21%, respectively) age ranges were significantly higher than obesity rates in the preschool age range. Thus, male and female youth have a much higher rate of obesity between the ages of 6 and 19 years than children ages 2–5. The rates of obesity jump quite a bit from the oldest youth age range (12–19) to the youngest adulthood age range (20–39). And the jump is significant for both males and females.

Both young adulthood males and females jump to an obesity rate of over 30 percent (30.3% and 34.4%, respectively), and both male and females in the middle-aged adulthood range hovered on either side of 40 percent (38.3% and 42.1%, respectively). Younger adult and middle-aged adult women had higher obesity rates than men in those age ranges; however, there was no identifiable difference between males and females in the older adulthood range. Thus, the differences between adult males and females overall seems to be accounted for by the fact that there are more obese young adult and middle-aged adult women than men. The highest rate of obesity among either sex was in the middle-aged adult range (38.3% for men and 42.1% for women), and the lowest rate for both sexes was in the young adulthood range (30.3% for men and 34.4% for women).

Race/Ethnicity

Race is an additional factor that can be considered when describing the BMI landscape in the United States. Reports indicate that the rise in obesity is found across all age groups and racial groups in the United States; however, certain racial groups show a greater increase in obesity than others.

The CDC classifies different groups by Hispanic and non-Hispanic origin. Thus, the categories used by the CDC to account for differences during the years 2011–2014 are Hispanic, non-Hispanic Asian, non-Hispanic black, and non-Hispanic white. During this time frame, the lowest rate of obesity was found among non-Hispanic Asian adults with an obesity rate of 11.7 percent and the highest rate was found among non-Hispanic black adults with a rate of 48.1 percent. Non-Hispanic white adults and Hispanic adults fell in-between these two groups with rates of 34.5 percent and 42.5 percent, respectively. The CDC reported that the differences between all groups are statistically significant, which means it is accurate to conclude that non-Hispanic Asians have the lowest obesity rate followed by non-Hispanic whites, Hispanics, and non-Hispanic blacks.

When breaking down racial and Hispanic origin obesity rates by sex, the order of rates from lowest to highest remained the same for women with non-Hispanic Asian women at a rate of 11.9 percent and non-Hispanic black women with a rate of 56.9 percent. The findings were different for men. While non-Hispanic Asian men had the lowest obesity rate at 11.2 percent, the highest rate was found among Hispanic men at a rate of 39 percent. Non-Hispanic white men and non-Hispanic black men had rates that were not meaningfully different (33.6% and 37.5%, respectively).

Overall, when comparing race and Hispanic origin by sex, differences were found only between non-Hispanic black women and men (56.9% and 37.5%, respectively) and Hispanic women and men (45.7% and 39%, respectively). This means that non-Hispanic Asian men and women and non-Hispanic white men and women essentially have the same obesity rate. Overall, the highest rate of obesity among race and Hispanic origin is found among non-Hispanic black women, and the lowest rate is found among non-Hispanic Asian adults regardless of sex.

When looking at the data by race and Hispanic origin for youth (ages 2–19), there are some similar trends. Non-Hispanic Asian youth had the lowest obesity rate (8.6%) followed by non-Hispanic white (14.7%), non-Hispanic black (19.5%), and Hispanic (21.9%) youth. Non-Hispanic white youth had obesity rates higher than non-Hispanic Asian youth and lower than non-Hispanic black youth and Hispanic youth. There is not, however, a meaningful difference between obesity rates of non-Hispanic black youth and Hispanic youth making both categories displaying the highest rate.

When looking at the youth data by sex, again there are similarities to the overall numbers. Among females non-Hispanic Asians had the lowest rate (5.3%) followed by non-Hispanic whites (15.1%), non-Hispanic black (20.7%), and Hispanics (21.4%). While non-Hispanic Asian females had the lowest rate of obesity followed by non-Hispanic whites, the difference between non-Hispanic black and Hispanic females was not significant meaning that both groups are considered to have the highest rate of obesity among female youth. With respect to young males the lowest rate again was found among non-Hispanic Asians at 11.8 percent, which was followed by non-Hispanic white males at a rate of 14.3 percent; however, this was not a meaningful difference and therefore these two groups comprise the lowest rate among young males. Non-Hispanic black males (18.4%) had a rate that was higher than the previous two groups but lower than Hispanic males (22.4%) who had a significantly higher rate than all other groups.

When comparing race and Hispanic origin among youth by sex the only meaningful difference was found between non-Hispanic Asian males and non-Hispanic Asian females with obesity rates of 11.8 percent and 5.3 percent, respectively. This means that among youth it can be concluded that the group with the absolute lowest obesity rate is non-Hispanic Asian females.

In aggregate, the obesity data based on race and Hispanic origin suggest that lower levels of obesity are most likely to be found among non-Hispanic Asian people regardless of age or sex. And people who are Hispanic or non-Hispanic black may have higher rates of obesity depending on sex or age.

Socioeconomic Status: Income Level

Socioeconomic status can be measured by income level or level of education. Education level is fairly straightforward to measure; however, measuring income level is a bit more complicated and is not based simply on how much money someone makes but how much they make in relation to the poverty threshold. In this section we will examine how income level is determined and what the rate of obesity is among the various income levels.

The poverty threshold (updated each year to reflect the degree of inflation that has occurred) as determine by the United States federal government is based on how large a family is, how many children the family has (not including foster children), and how old the head of household is. The poverty threshold does not vary geographically which means that as far as the federal government is concerned the poverty threshold for a family of any size is the same regardless of whether they live on the east coast, west coast, or in the north or south. The general description of each threshold (primarily based on family size) is that the dollar amount associated with each family size is thought to reflect what a family of that size needs; however, the U.S. Census Bureau which establishes these guidelines notes that local government aid programs may use different measures of poverty to account for what a family might need in a particular area of the country. Thus, a local government might conclude that a family may need more or less income to be considered impoverished than what the federal government suggests.

The term typically used to describe level of income is called the income-to-poverty ratio. This ratio is simply the amount of a family's total income divided by the poverty threshold for a family of that size. Using the U.S. Census Bureau's guidelines, for example, the 2016 poverty threshold for a family of four is $24,300. A family of four that brings in that exact amount of income or less is considered to be living in poverty. A family of four that brings in more than $24,300 is considered to be not living in poverty. For example, if a family of four has a total income in 2016 of $25,000 their income-to-poverty ratio would be 25,000/24,300 = 1.03 or 103 percent. Thus, this family is making 3 percent *more* than the poverty threshold, which means they are not considered to be living in poverty. They would, however, be considered a low-income family. A low-income family has an income-to-poverty ratio of less than 130 percent, which means that a hypothetical family of four living in poverty would have an income of less than $31,590.

The data on the prevalence of obesity based on income levels for children and adolescents ages 2–19 is available for the years 2005–2008. In a CDC data brief for these years, it was reported that overall rates of obesity declined as household income increased and that this trend held for both boys and girls. It did not hold, however, for race and Hispanic origin. Overall, of those who are obese in this age range, 24 percent live in a household that has an income-to-poverty ratio of 350 percent or higher, 38 percent live in households with an income-to-poverty ratio between 130 percent and 350 percent, and 38 percent live in households with an income-to-poverty ratio of below 130 percent which is the low-income category. Thus, although low-income families have a youth obesity rate of nearly 40 percent, this income level does not constitute the majority of obese children and adolescents.

For adults (ages 20 years and older) the trends are somewhat different. For men obesity rates are close to being the same at all income levels although rates are somewhat higher among higher income levels (income to poverty ratio of 350% or higher). This diverges from the rates among children which indicate that rates drop as income levels grow. The trends of obesity among women reflect those found among children: obesity levels decrease as income levels increase. Overall, among obese adults 41 percent live in households where the income is at or above an income-to-poverty ratio of 350 percent, 39 percent live in households with an income-to-poverty ratio between 130 percent and 350 percent, and 20 percent have an income-to-poverty ratio of less than 130 percent indicating that most adults who are obese, like their child and adolescent counterparts, do not live in low-income households.

Socioeconomic Status: Education Level

Education level is another way that socioeconomic status is measured. The U.S. government uses the following categories to indicate level of education: less than high school education, high school graduate, some college, and college graduate. To determine what education level a household has, the standards are applied only to the head of household. The head of household is defined as someone who is single or who has paid more than half the cost of maintaining the household for the year.

In a CDC data brief published in 2010, rates of obesity among children and adolescents (ages 2–19) were shown to increase at all education levels when comparing rates from data collected in the years 1988–1994 and 2005–2008. This data were broken down by sex revealing that the obesity rate among boys increased from 4.5 percent to 11.8 percent in households with a college degree, and in households with less than a high school education the rates among boys increased from 15.3 percent to 21.1 percent. For girls the trends were similar. Increases in obesity rates were 5.4 percent to 8.3 percent in households with a college degree, and 11.4 percent to 20.4 percent in households with less than a high school education. During both time frames, overall obesity rates were lower as level of education of the head of household increased.

During the time frames of 1988–1994 and 2007–2008 for adults (ages 20+ years), obesity rates increased at all levels of education. For men the increase was from 15.6 percent to 27.4 percent in households with a college graduate and 22.6 percent to 32.1 percent in households with less than a high school education. For women the trends were the same and revealed an increase from 15.3 percent to 23.4 percent among households with a college graduate and 31.7 percent to 42.1 percent for households with less than a high school education. Obesity rates increased among women as level of education decreased during both time frames. Whereas for men, the obesity rate was highest in households with some college education and lowest in households with a college graduate.

Although obesity rates are generally discussed in terms of rates by age, it is clear that when examining obesity rates using other demographic variables including sex, race and Hispanic origin, income level, and education level, only looking at age does not paint the clearest picture.

CULTURAL AND POLITICAL ISSUES

Attention given to the rates of obesity and consequences of associated health problems that have been linked to this body size has extended beyond the health-care arena. Advertising campaigns, public health policy, and school-based programs are all involved in expanding the message that larger body sizes need to be made smaller for the overall health and well-being of the nation.

Ad Campaigns

All over the world various groups and governmental agencies that have identified a problem with overweight or obesity have taken to implementing ad campaigns to warn against the dangers of obesity. The primary target of these efforts has been children. One of the most controversial ad campaigns was launched in 2012 in the state of Georgia. The 2012 effort was the start of a five-year-long campaign designed to combat childhood obesity. The campaign was called *Stop Sugarcoating It, Georgia* and consisted of billboards and television ads. Although similar ad campaigns have been produced in other regions of the United States and the United Kingdom, the ad campaign in Georgia garnered a lot of attention and sparked discussion and debate among laypeople and health-care professionals.

The ads in Georgia were designed by Children's Healthcare of Atlanta in response to an overweight and obesity rate of 40 percent among children statewide. One of their primary concerns was that they claimed around 75 percent of parents did not think there was a problem. Thus, the campaign was targeted toward the primary caretakers of children emphasizing the part they play in the size of their children's bodies. The ads depicted children of both sexes, various ages, and various races and ethnicities looking unhappy. All of the children in the ads were overweight or obese by BMI standards. Some of the taglines for the billboards included "It's hard to be little girl if you're not," and "Being fat takes the fun out of being a kid."

Data collected on the effectiveness of the campaign indicated that some parents have said the ads were effective in making them aware of a potential problem. The mother of a 15-year-old boy was quoted as saying that the ads caused her and her son to take action so he could reduce his weight, feel better about himself, and reduce bullying based on his weight. Critics of the ads, however, have pointed out that the ads themselves are not uplifting and can be construed as negative. Critics further indicated that the ads may backfire and have the opposite of the intended effect. They noted that if kids feel stigmatized for being overweight or obese as a result of ad campaigns like this children may then be more likely to experience lower mood and self-esteem, and may be more likely to engage in unhealthy behaviors such as overeating and eating foods may be high in sugar and/or fat content. Children's Healthcare has said that despite the backlash their ad campaign can be considered a success since the result was an increase in dialogue about childhood obesity which they noted was a primary aim of the campaign.

In the past few decades a new type of advertising called social marketing has developed to address concerns that affect society as a whole. Traditional marketing capitalizes on what the product is, how it will be priced, where it will be marketed, and how it is promoted. Social marketing is thought to be revolutionary in the sense that it includes groups of people referred to as stakeholders who provide input on how a particular product or program may be implemented. Stakeholders are people who would be directly impacted by any policies that may be put in place. In the case of overweight and obesity, stakeholders might include health-care providers, parents, and individuals who are themselves overweight or obese. The idea is that these stakeholders can provide insight into what will be effective, rather than having companies or agencies who do not understand the nature of the problem decide what will be done. For example, if an ad campaign like the one in Georgia had involved a group of people who were already overweight or obese and/or researchers who study the effects of messages targeting those who are overweight or obese, they may have heard about how such an ad campaign could negatively impact those it was intended to help. They may also have heard that focusing on changing behaviors so that they are healthier rather than focusing on the objective weight of an individual can lead to better overall health.

Several social marketing campaigns in the United Kingdom (e.g., *Change4Life*, *SnackRight*), France (*EPODE*), and the United States (*VERB*) have been specifically designed to address childhood obesity by focusing on making lifestyle changes and influencing environmental factors that may affect habits related to eating and physical activity. By incorporating input from stakeholders who will be directly impacted by such efforts, the programs not only have a greater chance of the campaigns being widely accepted among those they are purported to target but are also successful in terms of seeing changes in behaviors. Although more research is needed to determine the effectiveness of social marketing efforts, those involved in designing and implementing such campaigns believe the potential exists for them to be effective and sustainable.

Those who craft ad campaigns, whether they use traditional advertising strategies or the newer social marketing strategies, the focus is on trying to combat what they and others see as an epidemic and a crisis. Researchers, however, caution that ads and other efforts designed to address overweight and obesity should avoid content that contains a shaming or stigmatizing quality to them, which can contribute to overweight and obese children feeling worse about themselves. This can, in turn, result in an increase in unhealthy behaviors such as overeating and low motivation for physical activity which is precisely what many of the ad campaigns attempt to address. The recommendation is to focus not on the size of a person's body but on supporting behaviors that are known to improve one's overall health: eating a wide variety of foods sufficient to fuel the body, and engaging in regular physical activity.

School Policies

The ongoing discussion around the obesity epidemic and diseases associated with it, particularly among children, has resulted in not only advertisements targeted at children and those who raise them but also schools taking a more active role in assessing and informing children about their weight status.

At least one advertising campaign in the United States (i.e., Atlanta's *Stop Sugarcoating It, Georgia* campaign) has suggested that parents are either unaware of the dangers that have been connected to being overweight or obese, or do not think the dangers are real or that serious. Possibly as a result of this perceived lack of concern by parents, attention has been directed at schools to help in the fight against obesity by having school personnel measure students' height and weight so each child's BMI can be calculated (see Chapter 2 for how BMI is calculated). The results, often referred to as a BMI report card, are sent to the children's legal guardians with varying instructions on what to do with the information.

The first state in the United States to implement a program that included sending BMI report cards home to families was Arkansas in 2003. This was part of a larger program that also involved making changes to policies related to nutrition within the schools. In subsequent years additional states—around half of all states—have followed suit and include a school-based program for measuring children's BMIs and providing that information to parents or guardians.

Since these school-based programs have been implemented, controversy has swirled around them. Medical associations such as the American Academy of Pediatrics have stated that programs measuring BMI annually should be conducted, and the Institute of Medicine has specifically recommended that school is the right place for this. Part of the thinking is that taking these measurements in schools nearly ensures that the BMI of all children can be collected and tracked. Critics, however, have indicated that school-based programs can contribute to intensifying the stigma and bullying that many overweight and obese children already experience. For example, the process of weighing students is not always done in private. Additionally, others have indicated that most students know that they or their classmates are overweight suggesting that the assessment process is unnecessary. By giving more attention to something that most kids are already aware of, it is possible that an explicit focus on BMI gives the message that too high of a BMI is a problem to be corrected which makes overweight or obese students a sanctioned target of attention.

Two studies conducted in 2011 and 2015 concluded that school-based measurement of BMI has not been connected to an improvement in students' health. Since BMI is used as an indicator of one's health, the results mean that measuring BMI and providing this information to families has not resulted in lower BMIs. One conclusion drawn from the study in 2011 was not that the measurement of BMI is ineffective but that how parents have been notified was the problem. In addition, one of the leading international professional organizations on eating disorders, the Academy for Eating Disorders (AED), published a position statement in 2009 pointing to evidence that a focus on body shape and size and a valuing of thin bodies can lead to a drop in self-esteem, increase on body dissatisfaction, and an increase in dieting behavior. Although an increase in dieting may sound like behaviors designed to fix the obesity problem, the AED pointed to the growing evidence that weight-control practices (i.e., dieting) in children and adolescents is a predictor of later weight gain. Simply put, if a child or adolescent diets to lose weight it is safe to predict that they will ultimately gain weight—which is exactly the opposite of what school-based programs intend. The AED further pointed out that not much attention has been given to the effectiveness of obesity prevention programs aimed at youth. Other studies, however, have concluded that a focus on health rather than weight (implying that health and weight are not synonymous) may be more effective. The AED's position statement concludes with an extensive list of recommended guidelines for school- and community-based programs that includes the idea that the WHO's definition of health should be considered so that programs are not solely focused on the absence of disease but on the overall well-being of the individual as well.

Some school-based programs for measuring and reporting on students' BMIs have been discontinued; however, other states have determined that this process is worth continuing pointing to the obesity epidemic and the health dangers associated with it.

CDC and Public Health Policy

The Centers for Disease Control and Prevention (CDC), founded in 1946, is part of the U.S. Department of Health and Human Services and was originally called the Communicable Disease Center. It was located in the south because at that time this was the region of the United States that had the largest concentration of malaria transmission. Since the 1940s the CDC has expanded beyond disease transmission to include any threat to the health of the citizens of the United States.

At the time of this writing, the headline issue on the homepage of the CDC website was simply titled *Zika Virus,* which is a disease transmitted by mosquito and affects the development of unborn fetuses. Additional highlighted features on the homepage include information related to preventing the common cold, addressing prediabetes, preventing lead exposure, and vaccinating children. Typing "obesity" into the website's search bar yields a multitude of links on the CDC site that do not fit on one page. In fact, the CDC's focus on the weight of the nation's citizens is such that there is a division within the CDC devoted to the issue with the name Division of Nutrition, Physical Activity, and Obesity. The purpose of this division is to "maintain health and prevent chronic disease by promoting healthy eating and active living for Americans of all ages."

The division's Overweight & Obesity web page features links to obesity on *Data & Statistics, Adult Overweight & Obesity, Childhood Overweight & Obesity, Resources & Publications, Health Food Environments,* and *Strategies to Prevent Obesity.* There is also a link entitled *Healthy Weight* which links to information about managing weight via calories in and calories out, or in other words how much you eat compared to how much your body uses along with a link to a BMI calculator. The Overweight & Obesity webpage also features strategies for losing weight, weight loss success stories, strategies for preventing weight gain, and ideas for parents to help their children achieve and maintain a healthy weight. The message from the CDC seems clear: obesity is a chronic disease that requires the attention and resources of the nation's government and its citizens.

The American Medical Association officially declared obesity a disease in 2013 which dovetails with the CDC's emphasis on addressing the epidemic. The CDC is a significant driver of public health policy offering reports on things, such as: *Early Care and Education Policy Review*, *Healthy Communities: What Local Governments Can Do to Reduce and Prevent Obesity*, and *School Health Policy*.

As the primary agency of the government that looks at what are the most significant threats to the nation's health, the fact that the CDC has devoted significant resources to identifying who is obese and what can be done about it makes clear the notion that body size is something that can be too large. This has resulted in various policies and procedures designed to assist schools, local communities and governments, and health-care providers in reducing the rate of obesity.

Political Attitudes toward the Overweight and Obese

In the beginning of the 21st century, the CDC published a set of maps of the United States showing how the obesity rates had been rising dramatically over the previous years. This coupled with Surgeon General Richard Carmona's statement that declared the United States has an obesity crisis and identified it as an epidemic were likely contributing factors in making weight and the BMIs of the nation's citizens a political issue.

The declaration of overweight and obesity being an epidemic has resulted in the implementation of school-based programs designed to address obesity among children, position statements and guidelines from various professional and governmental organizations stating what should and should not be done to address obesity at any age, and the production of ad campaigns designed to ensure that this issue is not overlooked especially as it pertains to children. Former First Lady Michelle Obama leveraged her powerful position and developed a program called *Let's Move!* designed to address the "Epidemic of Childhood Obesity." Former President Bill Clinton has devoted resources to obesity prevention via his foundation called the *Clinton Foundation,* which is focused on developing collaborative efforts between stakeholders at all levels on issues that affect well-being and quality of life. Some have questioned whether or not something like BMI should be politicized; however, others have suggested that politicians are precisely the right people to address the overall increase in body size among those in the United States.

Rogan Kersh, a professor and provost in the Department of Politics and International Affairs at Wake Forest College, suggested in 2009 that despite all of the resources poured into the issue of obesity to develop clinical interventions there has been little if any change in the state of overweight and obesity in the United States. He concluded that given the ineffectiveness of current efforts it may be left to politicians to enact change. Not everyone agrees that politicizing such issues can be effective. Marion Nestle, a professor and chair in the Department of Nutrition and Food Studies at New York University, predicted in 2003 that what would need to happen nationwide to see a change in overweight and obesity would require significant changes in how food is grown and processed. She noted that changes of this magnitude would most certainly affect the bottom line of major food companies. She concluded that this type of "threat is one reason why food producers contribute generously to congressional campaigns." That type of influence, she further concludes, can prevent larger government sponsored programs to be effective.

To date there is no program that has demonstrated effectiveness in widespread *and* long-term decline in overweight and obesity. The explanation for this may be what many have suggested is the primary issue but has not garnered the attention it deserves: the environment in the United States is a perfect breeding ground for larger bodies. An article published in the *Lancet* in 2002 indicated that the toxic environment of the United States involves significant changes in the types of foods we consume (e.g., increase in fast food consumption, increase in child and parent directed marketing, increase in soft drink consumption), increasingly sedentary lifestyle (which researchers are now linking to higher mortality rates regardless of fitness level or weight), and what the authors refer to as "barriers to change," which include defunded physical education programs, schools needing to contract with corporate food services to save money, parents working longer hours leaving less time to prepare homemade meals, and so on. The authors concluded that no amount of funding for research, treatment, or prevention will yield an effective plan until the toxic environment of the country is addressed.

Some have contended that the health-care field's failure to cure overweight and obesity means that politicians should take over these efforts. Others have suggested that politicians are too heavily lobbied by representatives of food corporations making their involvement compromised at best. Others have suggested that politicians may need to be involved but only insofar as they can help make sweeping changes to how the society of the United States functions. Regardless of one's viewpoint it is clear that the size of U.S. citizens' bodies is political fodder. To date, however, politicians seem to have had as much influence on body size as others who have attempted positive change: very little.

Size Discrimination

Most readers probably know that there are many federally protected groups that are identifiable by a particular demographic characteristic, such as age, sex, race, disability, color, creed, national origin, or religion. This protection means that it is illegal to discriminate or harass someone based on any of these characteristics. Similarly, the U.S. Equal Employment Opportunity Commission (EEOC) protects certain groups based on things such as marital status, political affiliation, status as a parent, sexual orientation, and gender identity against employment discrimination. Many states in the United States have similar laws on the books to prevent discrimination, harassment, or improper employment practices. A demographic characteristic that is not legally protected at the federal level is weight or body size. This means that there is no protection under federal law for individuals experiencing discrimination or harassment based on their body size or weight. There are some states and local governments that have laws against discrimination based on weight or personal appearance but according to the Council on Size and Weight Discrimination, the list is quite small. A publication by the National Association to Advance Fat Acceptance indicates there are only six cities in the United States that have laws protecting against weight discrimination.

A document published in 2009 by Yale University's Rudd Center for Food Policy and Obesity entitled *Weight Bias: A Social Justice Issue* (Weight Bias Report) reported that weight bias can negatively impact an individual's medical and psychological well-being. They also reported that weight discrimination has resulted in a lower earning potential, less opportunities for being hired or promoted, and that this type of bias negatively impacts opportunities for academic advancement or achievement. The Weight Bias Report states that weight bias exists because many people believe that stigmatizing and shaming those who are overweight or obese will be a motivator for them to lose weight, and if these people fail to lose weight it is due to lack of discipline or willpower. The authors of the report also note that since the current culture sanctions weight bias, values thinness, puts all responsibility for body shape and size on the individual, and has a media that continuously depicts overweight and obese people in a negative way weight bias will not stop and will continue to adversely affect those who are overweight and obese.

Due to the pervasiveness of weight bias on the job, in health care and in schools, and the significant medical and psychological consequences as a result of this type of bias, the Weight Bias Report recommended that weight be included among other demographic markers that are covered by anti-discrimination laws at the federal, state, and local levels.

MEDICAL RESPONSE

As has been previously mentioned, health-care professionals play a significant role in identifying those who are obese or at risk for becoming obese as well as making recommendations for weight gain prevention or weight loss intervention. The primary forms of medical intervention for obesity include behavior management, medication therapy, and weight loss surgery.

Behavior Management

Behavior management refers generically to an approach to treatment that addresses what a person *does* (i.e., how they behave), and how those behaviors are helpful or harmful. When it comes to the focus on body size, behavior management strategies typically focus on helping individuals use strategies that are designed to promote weight loss or alternatively to prevent weight gain. In fact, the behavior management approach is typically recommended prior to the patient being prescribed a weight loss medication, and is required before bariatric surgery is considered.

Behavior management strategies are relatively simple and straightforward in theory. As has been discussed in previous sections, the prevailing assumption is that if someone cuts back on how much they eat and they eat less than their body needs to function throughout the day they will see weight loss. This holds true for implementing an exercise routine. If someone burns more calories than they consume in a day then they should eventually see weight loss. As has already been discussed in Chapter 2 in the section entitled "What control do we have over changing our BMI," there is far more to changing body shape and size than the simplistic notion of calories in and calories out. Regardless of the factors that affect weight loss, weight gain, or weight maintenance, the fact of the matter is when people attempt to lose weight they are most likely going to go on a diet.

While the primary definition for the term diet refers to what you eat on regular basis, "going on a diet" refers to changing what you eat on a regular basis for the purpose of changing your body shape or size. And, more often than not, the changes made involve food restriction of one type or another. Individuals may focus on restricting overall caloric intake or they may restrict or eliminate certain types of foods altogether. Foods that are often a target of diets are foods that contain high amounts of fat, refined sugar, or simply carbohydrates. Some people take a stab at making these changes on their own, whereas others consult specific diet plans such as The Paleo Diet®, the Atkins diet, Weight Watchers®, Jenny Craig®, clean eating, the Cookie Diet, and so on. Many people pay exorbitant amounts of money to purchase products or services that are intended to help them follow and stay on a particular diet. To put this in perspective, the diet or weight loss industry is an over $60 billion dollar a year industry and includes diet plans and products as well as health club memberships and medical interventions. Depending on what is included in this measurement, some have estimated that the costs may actually be over $500 billion. Either amount is enormous. What is perhaps even more shocking than how much we spend on weight loss is what happens (or does not happen) as a result of these expensive efforts.

Despite the sheer numbers of those who *want* to lose weight, who have been prescribed weight loss by their physicians, and spend thousands of dollars to reach a particular weight loss goal, over 95 percent of people who go on some diet to lose weight will gain it all back (and many will gain more than they lost to begin with). That means that dieting has a success rate of less than 5 percent. This further means that when a health-care provider prescribes behavior-based weight loss they are prescribing an intervention that is nearly guaranteed to result in failure (i.e., eventual weight gain).

The argument has been put forth by some that diets in fact do work. That a lot of people do lose weight when they go on a diet—which is true. The issue is in whether or not people can keep the weight off. As noted in the previous paragraph the vast majority do not. This is where a lot of shaming can come in. When someone gains the weight they lost they are often told in one form or another that it was because they didn't have strong enough willpower or self-control. Thus, the reason they regained the weight was because they were weak. Any discussion about the complexities of weight loss and weight gain (e.g., genetics, metabolism, history of weight cycling) are usually met with an insistence that for most people it is still a matter of willpower—if they want it badly enough they will work harder and lose the weight permanently.

Another issue related to the idea of weight loss for those who have been identified as having bodies that are too big is whether or not weight loss results in any health improvements. So independent of whether or not weight loss in the long term is even possible the question remains: does reducing body size lead to health benefits? The accumulation of studies pointing to the negative health outcomes for those who are obese also point to a reduction in these health issues when weight is lost. What is not always examined in these studies, however, is the magnitude of this impact on health benefits and protective factors.

Thus, despite being a commonly recommended intervention for the treatment of overweight and obesity, behavior management strategies have yet to be proven to be effective with regard to long-term weight loss. Additionally, the data suggesting health improvements are a result of weight loss have too many confounding variables (i.e., factors that were not studied but that may explain the results of the study) making the conclusions about the benefits of weight loss questionable.

Medication Therapy

In addition to behavioral weight loss recommendations (i.e., eat healthy and exercise), the two other forms of treatment medically recommended to address overweight and obesity are medication therapy (i.e., pharmacotherapy) and weight loss surgery (i.e., bariatric surgery). The initial determination for whether or not either medications or weight loss surgery are prescribed is based on BMI. Weight loss medications, for example, are prescribed to adults with a BMI of 30 or greater, or with a BMI of 27 or greater and an accompanying medical problem that is commonly associated with obesity. Medication therapy is not recommended for children under 12 years old and, in fact, there are no drugs approved for use in the United States in children younger than 12. Regardless of the age of the patient, these medications are typically prescribed in addition to, rather than in place of, behavior management strategies as discussed earlier. Experts indicate that medications may not work for everyone and that given the unpleasant side effects of many medications some may find that medication therapy is not an optimal intervention.

In general weight loss medications are designed to manipulate a person's hunger and fullness cues or to make the body's ability to absorb fat more difficult. The expectation is that along with changes to eating and physical activity the use of weight loss medications should help people lose around 10 percent of their body weight. Additional effects of these medications may include changes in blood sugar, blood pressure, and triglycerides. Improvements may also be noticed in terms of mobility and overall inflammation. For most people, most of the weight loss will occur during the first six months of using the medication. After that time weight loss typically slows down and in some cases individuals may start to regain what was lost.

There are several drugs approved by the Food and Drug Administration (FDA) for weight loss. Three approved drugs are recommended for longer-term use as measured in terms of months or years. There are also other medications designed to suppress one's appetite that are approved for short-term use and that are also controlled substances because of the danger of abuse. Only one drug is approved for children ages 12 and older; the remaining are approved for adults only.

Orlistat (prescribed as Xenical or over-the-counter as Alli) is approved for adults and is the only drug approved for children 12 years and older. This drug is designed to prevent fat from food from being absorbed by the body. Side effects of this medication include stomach pain, gas, diarrhea, and leakage of oily stools. Lorcaserin (Belviq) is only approved for adults and is designed to influence the neurotransmitter serotonin so that a patient feels full after eating small amounts of food and will therefore eat less overall. This drug can interact with other medications and should not be taken with other drugs that affect certain types of neurotransmitters. Side effects of this medication can include headaches and dizziness, tiredness, nausea, and constipation. Phentermine-topiramate (Qsymia) is for adults only and is a combination of two drugs. One drug acts by suppressing appetite and overall desire to eat, and the other makes one feel full and makes the taste of foods not as appealing. Side effects of this prescription include tingling, dizziness, change in taste, difficulty sleeping, and constipation. This medication can also cause birth defects and is not prescribed to pregnant women or women who plan to become pregnant.

The final group of medications has the potential for addiction and is therefore considered controlled substances. As such these medications are typically prescribed for shorter periods of time. As a group they act on the centers in the brain that affect appetite so that a patient taking them either feels not hungry or full. These medications include phentermine, bezphetamine, diethylpropion, and phendimetrazine and are sold under various other names. There are other medications that are prescribed for weight loss but are not approved by the FDA for this purpose. Prescription of medications to treat something other than what they are approved for is called off-label use. These medications are usually prescribed for something else (e.g., depression) but are sometimes prescribed to help promote weight loss.

Regardless of the medication prescribed, it is clear that these medications can result in some weight loss; however, since none of the medications are for permanent use, eventually the patient will have to stop taking the medication which means that if they have not changed eating and physical-activity-related behaviors, it is likely that whatever weight was lost will be regained—and even then as has been discussed already dieting and exercise are not the sole purveyors of weight loss and weight gain. In addition to side effects, many of which are unpleasant, these medications are designed to influence our body's hunger and satiety cues which means we are likely to eat less—possibly less than what our body requires to adequately function. When that occurs, our body has the ability to compensate for the lack of intake by slowing our metabolism the result of which is for the body to hang on to and store whatever food is eaten.

As with any medical intervention, it is important that those considering this form of treatment or who have been prescribed this form of treatment are fully informed of the likely effectiveness of the medication, what the common and uncommon side effects are, whether or not the prescription is being used off label, and if the medication may interact with other medications (prescription or over the counter including herbal supplements). They will also need to be sure that they are fully prepared for what happens once they stop taking the medication since none can be taken indefinitely. Only the person taking the medication can know if any possible benefits outweigh possible negatives.

Weight Loss Surgery

Weight loss surgery also known as bariatric surgery has been around since the 1960s. There are several different types of bariatric surgery, but they are only recommended for adults with a BMI of 40 or over, or a BMI of 35 or higher with an accompanying obesity-related health problem. Surgery can be recommended for children with slightly more strict criteria and will be discussed later in this section. Surgery is not, however, recommended for everyone who may fit the BMI and health-related criteria. Since bariatric surgery is designed to significantly alter the gastrointestinal system by rerouting it or removing a piece of it altogether, a potential patient should be adequately prepared for what the surgery can and cannot do for them, especially since not all procedures are reversible.

Although some people may see surgery as a quick or easy fix, medical professionals counsel patients that bariatric surgery is not a quick or easy fix and that the surgery alone will not address all factors that may have contributed to obesity. It is common and in many cases it is required that patients receive pre-bariatric surgery counseling to make sure they are good candidates psychologically for the procedure and that they are aware of the typical effects of the surgery. This type of assessment is usually done by a licensed psychologist who conducts a clinical interview and a formal psychological assessment. The clinical interview covers areas such as the patient's reasons for seeking surgery, their weight history and history of dieting, what their current eating behaviors are, and their understanding of the surgery itself as well as lifestyle changes they will have to make post-surgery. It is also common to include a discussion of social support the patient has had in the past and what they currently have, and their history of psychological disorders and treatment of those disorders. The psychological assessment portion of the process may involve a personality inventory designed to measure personality factors that might facilitate or interfere with the surgery.

Bariatric surgery is sometimes performed on youth; however, because a child or adolescent is still going through critical developmental processes in both the brain and the body, caution is recommended. To date there is not sufficient research on what effects bariatric surgery might have on the overall development of a child or adolescent. When bariatric surgery is considered for a child, there are conditions that should be met before considering this form of intervention. For example, it is recommended that the child has attempted to lose weight via other methods for at least 6 months without success. Additionally, the child should have a BMI of 40 or greater, should be 13 or older for girls or 15 or older for boys (it is likely they will have reached their adult height by that time), and they have a significant obesity-related health problem. Additionally, since these procedures are designed to alter (sometimes permanently) the functioning of the body's gastrointestinal system the decision to have bariatric surgery performed on a minor should require additional consideration as to its appropriateness.

Currently there are four forms of bariatric surgery that can be performed laparoscopically or by using an open approach. In laparoscopic surgery, small incisions are made through which surgical instruments and a small camera are inserted. This form of surgery requires less healing time and is likely to result in fewer post-surgical complications such as hernia. Most bariatric procedures are performed laparoscopically; however, not all patients are candidates for this form of surgery and may require open surgery, which involves a much larger incision to open up the body sufficiently enough to reveal the digestive system. The four forms of bariatric surgery most commonly performed in the United States are the adjustable gastric band (AGB), Roux-en-Y gastric bypass (RYGB), biliopancreatic diversion with a duodenal switch (BPD-DS), and vertical sleeve gastrectomy (VSG). The cost for all forms of bariatric surgery is significant at over $20,000 which may or may not be covered by insurance.

The adjustable gastric band (AGB) procedure decreases food intake by having a band placed around the top of the stomach making the opening from the throat to the stomach smaller than it is naturally. The size of the opening is adjusted based on the patient's needs by inflating or deflating a small balloon that is inside the band itself. The Roux-en-Y gastric bypass (RYGB) procedure also restricts food intake by creating a small pouch at the top of the stomach and bypassing the stomach, duodenum and upper intestine so that food is diverted directly to the small intestine. The bilio-pancreatic diversion with a duodenal switch (BPD-DS) involves removing a large portion of the stomach itself resulting in three effects. A patient will feel full sooner upon eating, food will be diverted around a significant portion of the small intestine, which reduces how much food is absorbed, and finally the digestive juices used to digest food and absorb calories are affected resulting in less food digested and absorbed. Finally, the vertical sleeve gastrectomy (VSG) decreases food intake as well as how much food is digested and absorbed by having a significant portion of the stomach removed resulting in a more tubular shaped section (similar in shape and diameter to the small intestine) or gastric sleeve.

There are numerous side effects that can occur or in some cases are likely to occur as a result of these procedures. Side effects from any surgical procedure can result in bleeding, infection, and blood clots. Due to the nature of bariatric surgery, there can be leaks from where intestines are sewn together and the patient may be more likely to experience diarrhea. Post-surgery, side effects that can occur as a result of these procedures include poor absorption of nutrients that can result in damage to the nervous system if not identified and treated properly. Additional side effects include hernia which is when part of an organ pushes through a weak muscle area, and strictures which occurs when the site where the intestines are joined narrows unintentionally.

The risks for bariatric procedures are significant since the gastrointestinal system is being altered from its original form (in some cases a part of the stomach is removed altogether). Thus, the importance of being fully informed of the benefits as well as all possible costs cannot be understated. Patients who choose this form of treatment have to closely monitor what and how much they eat and often have to adhere to a strict regimen of daily supplements to be sure the body is still getting all the nutrients it needs to function properly. Moreover, although bariatric surgery is cited as an effective treatment for morbid obesity, none of the procedures cure obesity. Thus, despite some weight loss, the amount lost is not always sufficient to remove someone from the obesity category, and the procedures themselves do not prevent weight gain from occurring post-surgery.

Therefore, significant weight loss is not guaranteed, and whatever weight loss does occur may or may not stay off.

One significant and irreversible cost associated with these procedures is death. Although the death rate is purported to be low and recommendations regarding bariatric surgery suggest that the "mortality rate should be less than 1%" at least one study that looked at the mortal rate among over 16,000 patients found that the rate post-surgery was 2 percent after 30 days, 2.8 percent after 90 days, and 4.6 percent after 1 year. Thus, the rate of death may be 2 times to over 4.5 times what it is purported that it should be.

Although there are various weight loss options that may be recommended by one's health-care provider, none have been shown to be a reliable method to achieve significant weight loss over the long term. Given the possible side effects and negative consequences of these interventions, it is recommended that any patient become fully informed of all potential risks, the likelihood that the procedure will help them meet their long-term goals, and the degree to which one may have to alter how they live their lives as a result of a procedure that may not be reversible.

CHAPTER 4

Consequences of How Overweight and Obese Are Treated by Society

In previous chapters readers have learned about which body shapes and sizes have been revered throughout the last century. We have also examined how body size is currently measured, evaluated, and how the degree of one's health is often linked to one's BMI. The focus on body size and BMI in particular has influenced ad campaigns designed to target overweight children and their parents, shaped how medical professionals intervene with their overweight or obese patients, and shaped public health care and school policies. This focus on BMI has also seen an accompanying trend in prejudice and discrimination against those with larger bodies.

The focus of this chapter is on a concept often referred to as "anti-fat bias." This bias simply refers to the idea that when an individual thinks about or sees a large or fat body they immediately have negative thoughts and feelings about not only the person's body but also the person's character. This chapter will examine how anti-fat bias may affect how individuals who are overweight or obese are viewed by health-care professionals and whether or not larger bodied people have access to the same services that those with smaller bodies have access to.

WHAT IS ANTI-FAT BIAS?

Anti-fat bias is one among many terms used to describe a particular way someone may view another person with a large, or fat, body. Other terms include weight stigma or stigma of obesity. A bias of any kind whether involving someone's body size, sex, skin color, religious affiliation, or any number of other ways in which we categorize people refers to holding a prejudice either for or against someone categorized a particular way. For example, we can be biased or prejudiced *in favor of* someone who has a particular religious affiliation. When this is the case we will automatically assume positive things about them and are more likely to give them the benefit of the doubt if there is any question about their behavior. By contrast, we can hold a bias or prejudice *against* someone who does not hold a particular religious affiliation and thus we automatically assume negative things about them while also assuming their guilt should there be any question about their behavior.

Whether the bias is in favor of or against someone, the end result is that the assumptions made about that person are made unfairly. Though most of us usually associate unfairness, in this context, with being prejudiced against someone it is equally unfair to be prejudiced for someone. In both instances, assumptions made are not based in fact or on direct experience with that person, but based on what we assume or think we know about them due to one particular characteristic. In this case: body size.

Examinations of anti-fat bias often include a discussion of its counterpart the pro-thin bias. Whereas someone holding an anti-fat bias would assume mostly negative things about someone with a larger body, someone with a pro-thin bias would assume mostly positive things about someone with a smaller or thin body. The two ideas are typically positively correlated. That is, the stronger someone's anti-fat bias is the stronger their pro-thin bias is with the reverse also true. Thus, if someone views fat bodies and the people who have them negatively then they are much more likely to overly value thinner bodies and the people who have them.

In the next section, we'll take a look at the degree to which anti-fat and pro-thin biases are present in health-care settings and the effects such biases can have on the patients who seek care from them.

MEDICAL CARE

By far the most research conducted in the area of anti-fat bias or the stigma of obesity has been among medical professionals. This focus likely has more to do with obesity and overweight being viewed as medical issues rather than there being a unique problem among medical care providers. Though the issue of whether or not professionals are biased against larger bodies can be studied easily enough through a dispassionate examination of data and statistics, the issue is decidedly an emotional one as well. No doubt readers are familiar with what has been called the war on obesity and anyone who regularly uses social media will have encountered stories of individuals with large bodies being made fun of, being discriminated against, and in some cases being assaulted simply for inhabiting a body that has been deemed to be too big. The following sections will examine the data on whether or not health-care professionals share the anti-fat bias that some in the U.S. seem to have adopted.

Is There a Bias among Health-Care Professionals?

Most researchers examining the idea of anti-fat bias among health-care professionals note that anti-fat bias exists in the culture at large and is therefore not exclusive to the health-care field. These researchers point to the idea that we are exposed to numerous messages not only warning us of the dangers associated with being fat but also implying or stating out right that individuals who are overweight or obese are lacking in positive personal characteristics as well. These researchers also note that health-care professionals are exposed to these same messages and therefore are not necessarily immune to their impact. Indeed, research in this area confirms that while anti-fat bias among health-care professionals is lower than that in the population at large it does exist and can have a negative impact on the patients they treat.

Anti-fat bias can be studied in a variety of ways; however, there are two common ways this concept is examined: explicit anti-fat bias and implicit anti-fat bias. Explicit anti-fat bias refers to consciously held beliefs that someone has about fat people. This means that if asked, they would readily acknowledge that they view overweight or obese individuals more negatively than thinner individuals—they are consciously aware of these beliefs. Measuring this is simple enough: one simply has to ask. This is usually done via a paper-and-pencil questionnaire and what is being measured is usually transparent (i.e., obvious to the person filling out the questionnaire). This raises an important question, however, in terms of the degree to which people who complete these questionnaires are answering truthfully. After all, despite the fact that an anti-fat bias seems to be common within the culture at large, not everyone will be comfortable readily admitting they have negative opinions about fat people, especially those who have pledged to care for their health and well-being. Thus, researchers have turned to implicit anti-fat bias as a way to get at what people really believe even if they don't want to admit it.

Implicit anti-fat bias involves tapping into strongly held beliefs that someone may not be consciously aware they have, or may not be willing to intentionally admit. The IAT or Implicit Association Test was developed by social psychologists, Anthony Greenwald and Mahzarin Banaji, who were interested in measuring just that. They developed a computer-based test that asks participants to categorize various descriptors. For example, the two categories may be "flowers" and "insects." Participants are first tasked with categorizing positive descriptors (e.g., excellent, joyful) with flowers and negative descriptors (e.g., horrible, nasty) with insects. When a particular descriptor is displayed on the screen they are to press the key on a keyboard that corresponds with either flowers or insects. So, if the word "excellent" is displayed then they need to press the key that corresponds with flowers, and if the word "horrible" is displayed then they are to press the insects key. The next phase is for participants to categorize the same descriptors, but this time the negative descriptors are to be categorized with flowers and the positive descriptors are to be categorized with insects (the reverse of round one). The assumption is that it will be easier for most people to correctly categorize the negative or positive descriptors with the category that they already associated with those descriptors. Since most people associate positive things with flowers and negative things with insects, the prediction would be that round one would be easier than round two. This is in fact what researchers find, and they measure this by reaction time. It takes people longer to match descriptors to the category that they do not already associate with that category—in this case flowers with words such as horrible and nasty, and insects with words such as excellent and joyful.

In the case of anti-fat bias, the IAT works the same way. The words "fat people" and "thin people" are the two categories under which either positive or negative descriptors must be categorized. Individuals who have an anti-fat bias will take longer to match positive descriptors such as "wonderful," "smart," or "motivated" under the fat people category and will more quickly match negative descriptors such as "horrible," "lazy," or "stupid" under the same category thus revealing an implicit or unconscious bias.

Research in this area with health-care professionals has revealed that although their bias is less than that found in the population at large, an anti-fat, pro-thin bias does seem to exist among health-care professionals. The researchers further concluded that when the bias did exist it was not contained just to fat bodies, but extended to the individuals themselves and how they were perceived by their health-care providers. This means that when health-care providers have an anti-fat bias they are not simply predisposed to think that the person is unhealthy, they are also likely to attribute characteristics such as lazy, stupid, and nasty to these patients. Holding such beliefs, even if they are not consciously held, has been shown to have important implications for the type and quality of care overweight and obese patients will receive.

Some efforts have been made to determine whether or not health-care providers in training can be prevented from holding an anti-fat bias in their work. One particular study published in 2013 examined the effectiveness of anti-stigma films on explicit and implicit biases. The films were developed by the Rudd Center for Food Policy and Obesity at Yale University. One film discussed myths and facts about weight and obesity, and the other discussed weight bias in health-care setting. Prior to viewing these films, students training to become either dieticians or medical doctors demonstrated implicit and explicit weight-related bias. After watching the two films, explicit anti-fat bias seemed to improve; however, implicit anti-fat bias did not. Researchers also noted that the reduction in explicit anti-fat bias did not last. They concluded that although the use of education-based films may be beneficial they suggested that more intervention is needed to sustain the diminished bias. One such possibility is to have participants discuss and examine the issues related to obesity and stigma in addition to watching the films.

Another study examined explicit and implicit bias among pre-professionals in the field of kinesiology and included a more experiential component to addressing anti-fat bias. Since students of kinesiology often work to become physical therapists or athletic trainers, they are often involved with patients/clients in terms of their exercise behaviors. There are many potential barriers to whether or not someone will engage in exercise (regardless of body shape and size) and the researchers noted that one such barrier is anti-fat bias. Kinesiology students enrolled in a tests and measurements course where required to engage in a service learning project that involved discussions and role-playing issues related to overweight and obesity. Results revealed a reduction in some characteristics related to explicit anti-fat bias, but there was no reduction in implicit anti-fat bias. The researchers concluded it is possible that implicit biases can be so deeply held that they may be resistant to change.

Although anti-fat bias prevention is a relatively new field of study, one group of authors reviewed what had been published in the area of reducing anti-fat prejudice to see if there were any notable trends. They examined all studies published as of 2010 regardless of whether or not the participants of the studies were health-care professionals or students. Their first conclusion was that there was very little published in this area (only 16 studies) which makes drawing conclusions about what works and what does not work to prevent anti-fat bias difficult at best. They also found that although some studies showed that changing what people think and know about the causes of obesity may be possible, changing the prejudice against fat people did not reliably change. Thus, even if people learn that the size of one's body has multiple causal factors and is not entirely within one's control, they will not necessarily demonstrate a reduction in anti-fat bias.

Additional research is clearly needed to more fully understand anti-fat bias and how it can be prevented. Current research shows that some aspects of anti-fat bias can be changed in those who hold it; however, findings suggest that for some people anti-fat bias is so strong and deeply held that it may be difficult to change.

Effects of Anti-Fat Bias on Treatment and Overall Well-Being

An assumption of studying and trying to prevent anti-fat bias is that the bias in and of itself is potentially harmful. This section examines what has been found in terms of quality and quantity of health-care services when health-care professionals have an anti-fat bias.

In 2010, Rebecca Puhl and Chelsea Heuer published a review of the research as it relates to weight stigma (i.e., anti-fat bias), how the pervasiveness of this prejudice may affect the health of individuals, and how it may threaten public health. They noted as others have before them that stigmatizing weight is often viewed as an effective intervention and prevention strategy. The belief among those that espouse this approach is that stigmatizing those who are overweight or obese will serve as a motivator for behavioral change. Puhl and Heuer noted, however, that as weight stigma has become more pervasive over the years there has not been an accompanying drop in rates of overweight or obesity and in fact those numbers have continued to climb.

In their review of studies focusing on the impact of weight stigma, they reported it is clear that individuals who experience weight stigma on a regular basis are more likely to have psychological and physical health problems. For example, weight stigma has been identified as being a risk factor for mood disorders such as major depression and some forms of anxiety. It is also connected to low self-esteem as well as body dissatisfaction. Some studies have connected weight stigma to an increase in behaviors that can be classified as disordered eating behaviors and for some these behaviors meet the criteria for a diagnosable eating disorder (e.g., anorexia nervosa, bulimia nervosa, or binge eating disorder).

Puhl and Heuer also examined the literature on weight stigma and its effect on physical health. They found that experiencing regular weight discrimination has been linked to changes in biochemistry that account for how body fat is accumulated and stored, and it has been linked to blood sugar intolerance. Thus, the more an individual experiences discrimination based on their weight, the more likely it is that their body will literally change how it metabolizes food and stores food byproducts. In their discussion of their findings, Puhl and Heuer point to the research establishing a link between pervasive forms of prejudice (e.g., racism) and the development of different forms of cancer, high blood pressure, and other cardiovascular problems. They suggest it is possible that regularly experiencing weight prejudice may have the same negative health effects.

Another way that anti-fat bias may be expressed is in the atmosphere of health-care clinics and offices themselves. Anti-fat bias may be reflected in the comfort of waiting rooms and the availability of medical equipment that can accommodate larger bodies. For example, some waiting rooms provide a variety of seating options that can accommodate any body size, whereas others may only offer seating that easily accommodates normal size bodies. Additionally, equipment such as regular sized blood pressure cuffs may not accommodate larger arms and thus this health measurement may not be attainable. In addition to being aware of how one interacts directly with people who are overweight or obese, those who are advocates of removing anti-fat bias from health-care settings recommend making sure that all aspects of a health-care facility can easily and comfortably accommodate any body size.

As noted above, researchers have suggested that anti-fat bias experienced on a daily basis is connected to a variety of negative health outcomes which ultimately might bring a patient to a health-care facility. Regardless of the reasons for an overweight or obese person's visit to a health-care provider, the quality and quantity of the care provided may facilitate or hinder the patient's overall well-being. Given the findings that experiencing an anti-fat bias may lead to negative health consequences and thus may be one reason a patient seeks assistance, researchers have turned their attention to what kind of health-care overweight and obese patients receive.

Puhl and Heuer found that providers treating patients who are obese spend less time with their patients and provide less health-related education. They also reported that patients indicate weight is usually identified as the cause of whatever has brought them to the provider—no matter what brought them to the office—and obese patients are less likely to obtain preventative care for things like cancer screenings. Phelan and colleagues found in 2015 that things have not changed since Puhl and Heuer examined the research in 2010.

Phelan's group found that a common bias some health-care providers have is that obese patients are lazy and are unlikely to follow treatment recommendations. This can then lead to less effective communication overall, and potentially less time spent with the patient educating them about their health. They also found that obese patients are likely to have their weight identified as the primary cause of whatever ails them which may mean these patients are less likely to receive diagnostic testing or hear about treatment interventions other than weight loss. They cited one study that found among patients whose primary symptom was shortness of breath, obese patients were advised to make lifestyle changes while their normal weight counterparts received medication.

Both Puhl and Heuer, and Phelan and colleagues concluded that patients who experience weight stigma in the health-care setting are likely to feel embarrassed and humiliated, which can lead to an overall drop in quality and quantity of care. The health-care professional himself or herself may not provide the same type of care that he or she would to a normal weight patient with the same symptoms. Additionally, however, the patient themselves may not fully process the information they are receiving due to experiencing high levels of stress at the office visit, which may result in difficulty concentrating and accurately processing information. The result is that patients who fear weight stigma in a health-care setting may be less likely to receive high quality care, and may be less likely to present for routine checkups and other preventative screenings the result of which can be that health issues go undiagnosed and untreated.

Researchers have found that weight stigma or anti-fat bias can be connected with negative health outcomes both psychologically and physically. They have also found that health-care professionals are not immune to anti-fat bias which may further exacerbate any health concerns their patients have. Research in the area of prevention of anti-fat bias in the health-care field is still quite young and there are currently no clear paths to identifying and preventing anti-fat bias from negatively impacting health-care received by overweight and obese patients.

Dangers of Using a One-Size-Fits-All Approach

The prevailing concern when it comes to overweight and obesity is that people who fall into these BMI categories are at greater risk for various diseases than those who do not have a BMI that classifies them as overweight or obese. As was also pointed out while these associations are repeatedly found in various scientific studies, it is important to note that the association or connection (also known as a correlation) between obesity and a particular disease does not mean that obesity is the cause of that disease. This is especially important in the sense that if we assume being obese or overweight is the cause of a particular disease then we will also assume that all people who fall within those BMI categories automatically have that particular disease or will eventually develop it. Thus, we will assume that anyone with an overweight or obese BMI is an unhealthy ticking time bomb for various debilitating diseases. We might also make the assumption that those who fall outside of those BMI categories (i.e., normal weight and underweight) are automatically healthy. This is, in fact, what can happen not only among the general population but also among health-care providers. Thus, there is evidence that the anti-fat bias may result in health care that falls below the accepted standard of care.

Those who study these issues warn that by applying the convention that larger bodies are unhealthy and smaller bodies are healthy the result may be to assume disease or disorder where there may not be one, or the absence of disease when there is in fact something to be diagnosed. They also note that an accompanying tendency may be to assume that the best treatment approach for the overweight or obese patient is weight loss when their thinner counterparts may receive treatment based less (or not at all) on weight and reflect treatment recommendations for the disease or disorder itself. This type of one-size-fits-all approach to health care may mean that there is a risk of treating overweight and obese individuals based on weight alone and recommending preventative weight loss for diseases that haven't yet been diagnosed. Additionally, there may be a risk of not screening for diseases among normal and underweight individuals because they are deemed to be already healthy since their weight is not too high.

ACCESS TO SERVICES

Access to services is not often a subject of debate or conversation when the issues of overweight and obesity are examined. For the most part, the conversation centers around the ideas of health and well-being with an emphasis on the potential physical consequences of having a larger body size. As the previous section noted, the issue of weight bias or weight stigma may be an important area of concern when considering the impact of being overweight or obese. There is a growing body of evidence to suggest that weight stigma is a significant factor in the overall health and well-being of someone who is overweight or obese. Since weight stigma may have a negative impact on one's overall health, it may also be important to consider the ways in which people with larger bodies have or do not have access to the same services as people with smaller bodies.

Airlines

Travel on airlines has seemingly become a lightning rod for myriad reactions to the place that larger bodies have in this mode of travel. Readers who have traveled by air have undoubtedly witnessed or themselves expressed disdain toward someone with a larger body who steps onto an airplane. Reactions to such a person can range from hoping that they will not be in the seat next to you to outright rage at the person for invading their space. Researchers Jennie Small and Candice Harris examined the experiences of passengers who are overweight or obese and posed the question: Whose responsibility is it to be sure larger bodies have an appropriate place on the airplane—the person themselves or the airline?

Drs. Small and Harris gathered information from a sizeable group of airlines on their policies and procedures (if any) when it comes to larger travelers, and they gathered information from online venues devoted to the issue of travel as an obese person. Their findings showed that the travelers themselves consistently expressed things such as feeling uncomfortable or embarrassed, and annoyed or fearful during their travel experiences as they knew they would likely be sitting in a seat that was too small for their body which would lead to their own discomfort. Small and Harris also revealed that those who are not overweight or obese seemed to be the ones who had more to say about obese travelers than the obese individuals themselves. They noted that there was decidedly an in-group, out-group mentality (i.e., us versus them) with complaints including the rights of nonobese travelers, feeling disgusted by having to sit directly next to someone who was obese, and the safety of passengers especially in an emergency.

Another issue these researchers examined is the fairness of cost. Small and Harris reported when examining the comments of nonobese travelers that some expressed concern for having to subsidize larger bodied passengers due to increased weight and noted that it was only fair that if they had to pay for an extra bag or a bag that weighed too much, then larger passengers should have to pay more to fly. Such passengers also stated that if both types of passengers pay the same amount for the same type of seat (e.g., coach class), but the larger person takes up part of the other person's seat, then their rights as a passenger have been impeded upon. When issues such as these occur some wonder whether or not the airlines themselves ought to intervene and establish protocols around body size and seat accommodation.

Small and Harris examined the policies and procedures of nearly 40 different airlines and found that only six had any explicit policies or guidelines about passenger size. Some airlines were specific in noting what could happen if a passenger could not reasonably fit into a standard seat. Things such as being able to put down the armrests or buckling the seatbelt were identified as necessary actions. If a passenger could not do one or both of these, then they would be required to purchase an extra seat or upgrade to a class with larger seats. Other airlines noted that if an obese passenger had not purchased an additional seat prior to the flight and there were no other seats available then the obese traveler may not be allowed to board the plane. Beyond such direct statements, Small and Harris found that the vast majority of the airlines had no policy about body size or had indirect statements that did not clearly state what would or would not happen should someone with a larger body size have difficulty fitting into the seat they purchased.

While clear and concise statements about body size and airline travel have the benefit of making it clear what needs to occur prior to or in the process of boarding a flight, the researchers argue that such polices may have the effect of sanctioning discrimination by passengers and crew members. That is, since passengers with larger bodies are explicitly singled out, passengers and crew may feel justified in any prejudice or discrimination toward an overweight or obese passenger. They further acknowledged that the rights, safety, and comfort of all passengers is important to consider, but noted that complaints lodged by non-obese passengers extended beyond what could be construed as reasonable concerns and entered the realm of disgust. They concluded that the strength of such opinions seemed to be fueled by the idea that obese people morally violate the expectation of thinness and health expected by contemporary society. Moreover, they concluded that comments turning toward disgust and hatred were likely accompanied by the notion that one's body size is fully within one's control. They suggested this may be the case since other passengers who have difficulty fitting (e.g., exceptionally tall individuals) into standard airlines seats are not met with the same furor since such passengers do not have control over things such as how long their legs are or how broad their shoulders are.

Small and Harris issued a call to action to the airline industry suggesting that since travelers' collective bodies are projected to get larger, not smaller, they literally cannot afford to ignore the disconnect between body size and seat size. Furthermore, the authors indicated that whatever action the airlines take, including developing clear polices where there currently are none, they need to do so in a way that does not bolster or incite the discrimination of larger bodied passengers. They suggest that a focus on being hospitable to all passengers ought to be primary and indicated that requiring the purchase of an additional seat or making someone sit in a seat so small that it can cause discomfort or injury does not make for a hospitable environment.

Though the issue of how to comfortably accommodate all body sizes during airline travel is far from solved, those who have examined this issue suggest any solution is likely to be complicated and ultimately may not be satisfying to all travelers.

Fitness and Exercise Facilities

Another service industry that individuals who are overweight or obese may wish to patronize is fitness and exercise facilities. Research in the area of fitness and exercise reveals that regular exercise regardless of body size can have myriad benefits on both mind and body. Those who are overweight or obese and who exercise routinely report, via online forums, that although they feel pressure from the culture at large to exercise in order to lose weight (or get healthy) they are often met with ridicule for actually doing what they think they are supposed to do or even want to do because of their body size. Some reported that they were ridiculed for the size of their body alone, others for the type of clothing they chose to wear (which is typically a similar type of clothing worn by other, smaller exercisers), or depending on the method of exercise they may be ridiculed for moving their body in inappropriate ways despite the fact that their smaller bodied counterparts have not received the same admonitions. The possibility of experiencing these types of interactions in person can be seen as barriers to using exercise and fitness facilities. Those who make it to a facility often have their fears confirmed when they interact not only with other exercisers but fitness professionals as well.

A study conducted by Noelle Robertson and Reena Vohora in 2008 revealed that an anti-fat bias was held by both regular exercisers and fitness professionals. They measured the degree of explicit anti-fat bias (bias that the exercisers and professionals are aware of in themselves) and implicit anti-fat bias (bias that they are not aware of in themselves). The researchers found results similar to other studies examining implicit anti-fat bias, but found that the explicit anti-fat bias was stronger in their study. Measures of explicit anti-fat bias are often affected by the desire of people to not appear bad or endorse socially unacceptable ideas. Thus, for many studies this means that people are less likely to consciously admit to viewing obese people more negatively than thin people. Robertson and

Vohora found, however, that the explicit anti-fat bias was strong enough among those who completed their study that fat people were rated much more negatively than thin people on things such as degree of motivation and laziness, and overall goodness as a human being. They also found that among regular exercisers, those who had never been overweight held a stronger anti-fat bias than those who had previously been overweight. Additionally, a strong anti-fat bias was held among fitness professionals who believed that body size is under that person's control which is consistent with the results of other studies.

Although Robertson and Vohora did not measure the manner in which regular exercisers and fitness professional interacted with obese patrons, they noted that research examining bias based on other criteria (e.g., race, mental health) has shown that when someone holds a bias against a particular group their interactions with someone from a member of that group will be affected, usually negatively. Thus, these researchers concluded that having an anti-fat bias would be no different. Other researchers have also found that an anti-fat bias exits among some fitness professionals and have further noted that the prevailing attitude toward overweight or obese exercisers is that they are lazy, do not have self-discipline, are annoying, and will not comply with recommendations. It is possible that when a fitness professional holds such opinions they may interact differently with an overweight or obese exerciser than how they would interact with someone who is not overweight or obese. Regardless of the degree to which a fitness professional has an anti-fat bias, those who have studied this issue agree that training fitness professionals to better understand the nature of obesity and related issues is important for them to be more effective with this population of exercisers. Moreover, it may be important for overweight and obese exercisers to find fitness facilities that not only support all levels of fitness but also all body sizes.

Medical Services

As discussed in the section on bias in health-care, professionals in health-care can have an anti-fat bias toward patients who are overweight or obese. In addition to the impact this bias may have on patient care (e.g., less time spent with obese patients, more likely to prescribe weight loss rather than other interventions), it can also affect whether or not an overweight or obese patient will seek services they may need.

Negative attitudes toward obese patients are reportedly not new. In the late 1960s, a study was published that reflected a negative bias toward larger bodied patients similar to those expressed in contemporary research studies. Additionally, this decades-old study revealed that some physicians stated outright that they would rather not have an obese person as a patient and if they did their expectation was one of failure on the part of the patient. Similar finding have been reported in the field of nursing and among dieticians.

Related to concerns about how an overweight or obese patient may or may not follow through with medical recommendations is a concern that overweight and obese people have more medical costs than others which can be passed along to others in the form of increases in insurance premiums. There are studies that show higher health-care costs associated with obese patients. Critics of such findings indicate that these studies do not to take into consideration things such as failure to get routing medical care and preventative screenings, which have been associated with experiencing an anti-fat bias. By not seeing one's physician regularly and by not getting preventative screenings (e.g., breast cancer, gynecologic exams), it is possible that the higher health-care costs have less to do with more health problems per se and more to do with delayed care. Delayed care may result in the emergence of pathology that could have been prevented and/or successfully treated in its early stages. Some have also suggested that higher health-care costs among overweight and obese patients may be a result of repeated but unsuccessful efforts to lose weight. Weight cycling or yo-yo dieting has been found to result in more medical problems than if the person had not attempted to lose weight to begin with.

Thus, lack of access to medical services may not be due to issues such as discomfort in waiting room seating—although this can be an issue in some waiting rooms—and more to do with a reluctance to set foot in a facility where the expectation is that the patient will be met with a negative attitude at best and discrimination at worst. Of course, many health-care providers treat overweight and obese patients with the kindness and respect that any patient deserves; however, if a patient is new to a practice they do not know what to expect. Their sensitivity to anything that makes them feel unwelcomed and undervalued may be particularly heightened should they have previously experienced anti-fat bias in another health-care setting.

Other Public Services

Obesity is not currently a protected class in terms of discrimination. That is, when laws exist regulating prejudice and discrimination of particular groups of people (e.g., groups based on race, ethnicity, religious affiliation, or sexual orientation), obesity is not among the groups listed. Despite this, some individuals believe that body size should be a protected class and have sued various companies due to discrimination based on their body size. When a lawsuit has been filed, the primary complaint often revolves around inadequate accommodations with respect to seating. In addition to airlines, as discussed in a previous section, other services such as restaurants, buses, and movie theaters have been sued for either not providing adequate seating or expecting that an additional seat needed to be purchased to accommodate one's body size. The lawsuits have had varying degrees of success; however, such suits as well as anecdotal information on public online forums suggest that many public services may not be aware of or care about the comfort of larger bodied patrons thus increasing the likelihood that an overweight or obese person may not access these services.

Education

There is a growing research base examining absenteeism among children and teens who are normal weight to obese. Findings consistently show that obese children are significantly more likely to miss school than their normal weight counterparts. Additional studies show that when in school obese children are more likely to underperform in comparison to their normal weight peers. They have also been found to have more detentions, a higher rate of tardiness, and less participation in athletics.

Often the conclusion from these studies is that interventions need to be designed or amended to include a focus on helping obese children perform better, and maintain regular and on-time attendance. Although this is not necessarily an incorrect conclusion to draw from the research, critics of this approach suggest that these studies did not look at the degree to which the obese children were experiencing anti-fat bias, which may directly affect whether or not a child attends school. It is possible, therefore, that the reason for an increase in absenteeism and a decrease in school performance is not based on obesity per se but on the prejudice and discrimination obese students experience as a result of anti-fat bias. Thus, some researchers have recommended focusing on interventions and prevention efforts targeting anti-fat bias among students and school personnel. Such efforts may result in a reduction in anti-fat bias which may have the effect of improvement in obese children's engagement with their education and extracurricular activities.

EFFECTS OF CULTURAL AND POLITICAL ATTITUDES

Weight stigma, weight bias, and anti-fat bias all point to a particular set of beliefs when it comes to particular body sizes and the people who have them. The bias is that larger bodies or fat bodies are unhealthy, unappealing, and those who have them should do everything they can to make their bodies smaller. Those who hold this type of bias also believe that people with smaller (i.e., thin or muscular) bodies are healthy, appealing, and that those who have that type of body should do everything they can to keep their body exactly the way it is. While it is true that some people who are overweight or obese are unhealthy and some people who are thin or muscular are healthy, the reverse is also true. Research examining the connection between being fat, and disease and mortality rates have found that there is a connection among these variables; however, many researchers point out that this connection does not determine whether or not overweight or obesity is the cause of particular disease or of an early death. Critics of studies that conclude obesity is the cause of these negative outcomes indicate that these studies often omit factors such as stress, access to health care, and other variables that are connected to the same diseases that obesity is. Maintaining that obesity is the cause of disease and death can lead to the perspective that society in general should do whatever it takes to motivate overweight and obese people to lose weight. One type of motivator that is often used is shaming. The idea is that if people feel shame about some aspect of themselves they will be motivated to make a change. Research has shown, however, that shame and ridicule are not effective motivators for most behavior change including weight loss. The research has shown that shame and ridicule can have negative health effects.

Psychological Effects

A study published in 2009 examined the effects of weight discrimination on psychological disorders. The researchers recruited over 20,000 overweight and obese adults who were part of the National Epidemiologic Survey on Alcohol and Related Conditions. They measured the degree to which these individuals perceived that they have experienced weight discrimination. Participants were asked how often they were prevented from or felt like they could not do something because of their weight. Included were such things as not getting health-care or health insurance, being discriminated against by a health-care provider, experiencing discrimination in public, discrimination at work, at school, in a training program, or discrimination in any other setting or situation. Participants also completed measures to assess their degree of mood and anxiety disorders, substance use disorders, degree of stress, and presence of social support. The results of this study suggested that more than 50 percent of those who perceived themselves as overweight or obese and who experienced weight-related discrimination met the diagnostic criteria for at least one psychiatric disorder (e.g., a mood disorder, an anxiety disorder, a substance use disorder). The analysis of the data revealed that stress itself was the contributing factor for these diagnoses and that the presence of social support (having good support from others in one's life) did not protect these adults from the effects of perceived weight discrimination. The conclusion drawn was that when people believe they are being discriminated against because of their weight they may be more likely to also experience a psychological disorder regardless of how much support they may have from friends and family.

Additional studies examining how weight stigma may impact overweight and obese individuals support the findings of this national study. Other researchers have concluded that weight stigma can be considered a public health issue when it comes to overall health including psychological health. Experiencing weight stigma in and of itself is considered a risk factor in the development of clinical depression. Other studies report that self-esteem drops when someone experiences weight stigma, and low self-esteem itself has been connected to problems in psychological and physical well-being. When controlling for factors such as when someone became obese, how old they were, what their BMI was, and if they were male or female, researchers found that an increase in mental health issues was not explained by the weight itself or any of these other factors. Rather, the variable that explained the inordinate rate of mental health issues among those who were obese was weight stigma. Recommendations based on such findings include the idea that any policies developed around addressing overweight and obesity must also include addressing weight stigma and anti-fat bias.

Although in some studies, social support has not been found to be important enough to counteract the effects of weight stigma, other studies have found that using other coping strategies to mediate the impact of weight stigma may be effective. When people use effective coping strategies to deal with weight stigma they are less likely to experience distress or a drop in psychological well-being. Many coping strategies are not universal meaning that what works for one person may not work for another. Additionally, in some cases men and women benefit from different types of coping strategies. For example, women who engaged in strategies such as positive self-talk and seeking support from friends and family experienced less psychological distress. Men seemed to benefit from adopting an attitude of self-acceptance in the face of weight stigma, whereas dealing with weight stigma by avoiding it or engaging in negative-self talk resulted in lower self-esteem. The effectiveness of coping strategies varies from one person to the next regardless of gender; however, it seems to be that when an effective strategy is found for an individual person it may be possible to combat the deleterious effects of weight stigma.

Physical Health

The link between weight stigma and negative physical health indices is not as well established as the link with a decline in psychological health. However, given the inextricable link between the mind and body, researchers have suggested that the connection likely exists. Thus, a decline in psychological well-being may lead to a decline in physical well-being as well. What does seem to have been identified in the connection between weight stigma and physical health is the impact weight stigma may have on eating behaviors and physical activity. That is, experiencing weight stigma may be connected with a decline in healthy eating and healthy physical activity.

With respect to eating behaviors and weight stigma, the focus has been on binge eating behavior. When considered in the context of an eating disorder (i.e., binge eating disorder or bulimia nervosa) binge eating is defined as eating a large quantity of food in a relatively short period of time. Although this is not a terribly precise definition, an additional caveat is that in the context of a binge most people would agree that a lot of food was consumed relatively quickly. In one study of over 1,000 women examining factors related to binge eating behavior, what contributed to binge eating episodes was not only the perceived experience of weight stigma but also internalizing this belief. Internalizing a belief refers to taking on a belief as your own. In this case, the women in this study who internalized ideas related to weight stigma +would themselves believe that larger bodies (i.e., their own body) are unappealing and unhealthy. When this belief was internalized they were found to be more likely to engage in binge eating behaviors. Despite the fact that the women in this study were also members of an organization focused on weight loss support, if the women believed their bodies were unacceptable as is, they were more likely to engage in problematic eating patterns (i.e., binge eating), which would in turn lead to weight gain. Findings from other studies have confirmed that exposure to weight stigma can be associated with a formal diagnosis of binge eating disorder, binge eating, or eating restraint (i.e., significant reduction in caloric intake), and in some cases purging (e.g., self-induced vomiting, laxative abuse) behaviors.

Studies that have explicitly examined the connection between amount of physical activity and weight stigma have predominantly been conducted with children. Those studies report that children who experience weight stigma engage in less physical activity or avoid physical activity altogether compared to those who do not experience weight stigma. One study of adults found an indirect relationship between weight stigma and physical activity. Among a modest sample of college students researchers found that motivation to avoid physical activity was connected with experiencing weight stigma, and motivation to avoid was connected with less frequent exercise. Although these findings collectively indicate that experiencing weight stigma may negatively affect amount of physical activity, additional research in this area would help to clarify the nature of the connection between weight stigma and exercise behaviors at all ages and at various weights.

In terms of specific medical issues, one bodily system that may be negatively affected by experiencing weight stigma is the cardiovascular system. One study conducted with children seems to have identified a connection. Children in this study who experienced stigma based on their appearance were more likely to have unhealthy blood pressures. Although an important mitigating factor for unhealthy blood pressure is life stress in general, researchers have postulated that experiencing weight- and appearance-based stigma is a highly stressful experience in and of itself. Since chronic stress is routinely connected to various illnesses including high blood pressure, it is possible that weight- and appearance-based stigma is stressful enough to have such an impact. The connection between stigma-induced stress and health markers such as cardiovascular problems and glucose intolerance has been well documented when the stress in question is induced via racism. It is possible then that the same strong connection between stress as a result of weight stigma and poor physical health exists. More research is needed however to more fully test this hypothesis.

The research in the area of weight stigma and physical health is far from definitive. There do, however, seem to be some trends suggesting that experiencing weight stigma may have a negative effect of physical health.

Internalization of Weight Stigma

A final consideration when discussing weight stigma is the degree to which the stigma is internalized. This idea has been mentioned previously; however, internalized weight stigma refers to the idea that the person who is on the receiving end of weight stigma from others internalizes the stigma and makes it their own. That is, they have weight stigma themselves and view bodies that are too big in a negative way, including their own.

A study conducted in 2004 by researchers from Yale University and the University of Pennsylvania found that people who were overweight themselves tended to have negative views of people in general who were considered overweight or obese. The authors noted that this is a unique finding as other groups that were on the receiving of bias and discrimination (e.g., race and sex) were not found to devalue members of their own group. In fact, they tended to view other members of their racial or gender group more favorably. The authors of this study suggested that overweight people who devalue members of their own group when members of other minority groups do not do the same is due in part to the prevailing belief that one's weight is under one's control. Therefore, if someone is overweight or obese they may also believe it is well within their ability to lose weight—they just have to try harder and be more motivated. If they remain overweight or obese then they consider themselves to be lazy, unmotivated, and bad. Additionally, since may people go on diets to lose weight but fail to keep the weight off, this confirms for them the idea that they simply do not have enough willpower or are too lazy to keep it off. Thus, members of this particular group perceive all of this a confirmation that they are bad or deserve to be viewed negatively by themselves and others.

A study conducted in 2016 found that weight bias internalization is an important factor when attempting to understand the impact of weight bias itself on eating behaviors and psychological distress. The authors of this study concluded that weight bias internalization can be considered a specific target of psychological intervention—rather than or in addition to the eating behaviors and psychological distress themselves. The authors further suggested that those in the position of making health policy ought to focus efforts and resources toward abolishing weight stigma via programming aimed at workplace, health-care, and school-based settings. By attacking weight stigma at the level of public health initiatives, the impact of weight stigma may be lessened. The idea would be that if the culture at large held a neutral or less negative view of overweight and obese bodies, then those who are overweight or obese would be less likely to internalize this stigma. They would not see themselves as deserving of bad treatment and ultimately may not experience the negative impact on their overall health.

Overall, research in the area of anti-fat bias has demonstrated that not only is it found among the average citizen as well as health-care professionals but that when someone experiences this form of bias there are associated negative consequences for their overall physical and psychological well-being. Some researchers have suggested that prevention efforts related to obesity ought not to target obesity itself but the negative bias people have toward obese people as well as the tendency for obese people to internalize this bias thereby viewing obesity just as negatively as others do.

CHAPTER 5

Health at Every Size®

The previous chapters have examined the facts related to BMI, obesity, and health, and have challenged widely held beliefs about the connection between body size and overall health. Additionally, the notions of anti-fat bias and weight stigma have been discussed and were revealed to be present among health-care providers and among service industry personnel. Additional research examining the impact of experiencing prejudice and discrimination based on body size has shown that one's physical and psychological health may be negatively affected as a result.

A growing body of literature has suggested that trying to change one's body size is not only not entirely within our control, but engaging in a cycle of weight loss and weight gain can result in greater health problems than if someone had not tried to lose weight to begin with. A parallel body of literature that continues to reveal similar results has shown that engaging in healthy behaviors such as eating as healthy as possible (without severely limiting calories or eliminating food groups or food types) and engaging in moderate and regular exercise has health benefits for people regardless of whether or not someone loses weight. Thus, someone who regularly engages in healthy behaviors will be healthier regardless of their body size and regardless of weight loss. One particular movement or approach to living espouses the belief that health is possible at any size when one embraces a focus on health and lets go of the focus on weight; it has become a movement among some laypeople and health-care professionals. This chapter provides a brief background and synopsis of the Health At Every Size® (HAES®) approach and what science has to say about it. Concerns about this approach will also be addressed.

What Is the History of Health at Every Size®?

In her book entitled *Health at Every Size: The Surprising Truth about Your Weight,* author Dr. Linda Bacon described how she pursued weight loss throughout her life with the hope of changing her life. She described how her experiences were similar to those she studied and with whom she worked: a struggle to maintain one diet regimen after another and not being able to sustain any of them. The result for Dr. Bacon was an increase in weight and a decrease in self-esteem, which eventually prompted her to learn as much as possible to figure out why she and so many others had been unable to lose and maintain weight loss.

Dr. Bacon initially earned a master's degree in psychotherapy during which time she learned about the psychology of eating disorders and body image issues. She stated that through her studies she learned that psychology alone did not account for the challenges human beings have with weight regulation. She then pursued a master's degree in exercise science where she specialized in metabolism. Finally, she earned her doctoral degree in physiology where she studied nutrition and weight regulation. The conclusion she drew from her multidisciplinary studies was that there was so much more to weight regulation than was commonly or publicly known. Moreover, she reported feeling very differently about herself, her body, food, and physical activity noting that she found pleasure again in things that had become a chore or were outright painful as a result of her prior obsession with weight loss and maintenance. The culmination of her personal and educational journeys was the publication of her book in 2008.

At the start of her book, Dr. Bacon notes that it is not a weight loss or diet book. Rather, she states it is a book intended to help readers turn away from an emphasis on weight toward an emphasis on health. In addition to the notion of ending dieting, she also tells readers that the book is intended to help them stop fighting with and hating their bodies for not looking the right way. Dr. Bacon tackles various myths about weight loss and weight maintenance and presents scientific evidence supporting her ideas. She then takes readers through the HAES® approach and explain how readers can implement the approach in their lives.

The HAES Approach and Its Major Tenets

Simply put, the HAES® approach takes the perspective that one's weight is not important when it comes to health and well-being—a view that is not shared by all health-care providers. Dr. Bacon contends that what matters is how one treats one's body. The idea is that when people engage in healthy behaviors they will improve their health, regardless of what size their body is. By taking this approach Dr. Bacon has attempted to disentangle the connection between weight and health by stating that one's weight is not an indicator of one's health despite the current cultural beliefs and health-care standards suggesting that a smaller body is a healthier body. She has rejected the assumption made by many people including health-care professionals that if you have a relatively normal weight body (typically measured using BMI) then you are healthy, and if your body weight and size are larger than normal then you are either already unhealthy or will become unhealthy in time.

The HAES® approach indicates that each body is designed to maintain its own healthy weight which is regulated in part by internal cues that let us know when we are hungry and when we are full. The idea is that a weight that is healthy for one person may not be healthy for another. Additionally, Dr. Bacon described how and why our bodies resist weight loss and what happens to our respective metabolisms if we engage in yo-yo dieting and/or restrict our food intake for an extended period of time. The approach also points to problems with respect to food politics (i.e., which foods are good and which foods are bad) and fat politics (i.e., larger bodies are a problem that need to be dealt with), both of which, she contends, further contribute to problematic eating and exercise behaviors that ultimately result in weight gain and poor overall health for many people. The HAES® approach encourages readers to push such cultural and sociopolitical issues aside and to reconnect with themselves and their body so that they relearn to nourish and appreciate their body regardless of what size it is. This, Dr. Bacon says, will result in improved physical and psychological health.

The first part of the approach is designed to help readers learn to love, appreciate, and respect themselves exactly as they are, which she notes can be particularly difficult when those around us are consistently giving us messages that the way our body looks is not okay. The HAES® approach provides examples readers can use to combat messages from friends, family, and the culture at large indicating that the only way to be healthy is to lose weight. This approach, for example, indicates that a shame-based approach is ineffective and can result in feeling both physically and psychologically worse. Those who wish to enact this approach are encouraged to let go of the fantasy that the only way to be happier, get a better job, date the person you want to, and so on, is to become thin. Instead, readers are challenged to engage in the things necessary to actually be happy now, to position one's self to get a good job or dating partner now rather than buying to the idea that weight loss is a necessary initial step. Other ideas of the first part of the HAES® approach include understanding what myths about obesity one has internalized, understanding what is personally motivating when it comes to weight, listening for negative self-talk, and interacting with others who can be supportive of your efforts even if it means they, too, have to learn about the HAES® approach. There are other tasks in this first section, but the overall theme is to more fully develop an awareness of one's self with respect to weight and size, to identify and resist the cultural and other pressures to be a particular size, and to learn to accept one's self as is without a focus on weight loss.

The second part of the HAES® approach is entitled *Take Care of Your Hungers*. This segment focuses specifically on food and hunger. Dr. Bacon notes that by fully listening to ourselves and our bodies we have everything we need to make healthy choices. She does not espouse the idea that certain foods should be off limits (unless of course there is a diagnosed medical reason, such as diabetes or celiac disease, to avoid or eliminate particular foods). Rather, she suggests that when we have learned to love and accept ourselves as we are, and we learn what motivates us we are better able to occasionally eat foods that are often off limits on various diet plans (e.g., sweets, carbohydrates, fats). She also indicates that we will be more effective at eating a variety of foods when we decide that what we need is to fuel our body so that it does what we want it to do. Dr. Bacon states that people who are able to do this will also be able to choose not to eat food such as pizza or ice cream simply because they are not hungry at all or hungry for that particular food. She clarifies that in such situations the decision is not rule based, it is not forced, it is simply an acknowledgment and recognition of what one's body wants or needs at that particular moment. The result of taking this approach is reportedly that by being able to interact with food in this way, we no longer have to declare that certain foods can never be eaten again only to find ourselves gorging on that particular food days or weeks later. Dr. Bacon concludes that foods normally off limits on most diets can and will be eaten because we have shifted our perspective from being at war with our body to being in cooperation with it and having a desire to care for it which involves eating a variety of foods and not living in a state of deprivation.

This section specifically encourages people to learn to more fully engage with their food by savoring things like taste and texture so that eating becomes a more pleasurable experience; to pay attention to yourself while you're eating so that you don't miss your satiety cues because you are so wrapped up in a movie or television show; to learn how to determine when you are full and when you are hungry (cues that are often ignored or that go unnoticed by many); and how to manage eating for the purpose of dealing with a particular feeling—often referred to as emotional eating. Dr. Bacon suggests that by paying attention to food and eating in these ways we will learn to trust ourselves and our bodies to know what to eat and when. We will learn to trust ourselves to eat in a healthy and enjoyable way.

The next element of the HAES® approach is referred to as *Live Well* and involves engaging in behaviors that further facilitate a healthy mind and body. Dr. Bacon reminds readers in the beginning of this section that although the book and approach are not focused on weight loss, many of the suggestions in this section are commensurate with maintaining a healthy weight. Maintaining a healthy weight, is clarified as not to be confused with weight loss per se, or with achieving a particular BMI, but with maintaining whatever weight is healthy based on one's particular body, age, and genetics. The various recommendations in this part of the approach include engaging in regular physical activity—but only engaging in activities that you find enjoyable or are willing to do and only as often as you're willing to do them. Dr. Bacon suggests that formally planning workout days and times does not work for everyone and indicates that another approach is to find ways to easily incorporate more movement into your daily life. This section also includes paying attention to nutritional intake including how food is processed, the benefits of eating a lot of plant-based foods, and eating a variety of food that is enjoyable to eat. She also notes that gaining a sense of overall health and well-being involves getting enough sleep and learning how to effectively manage stress via relaxation.

The final section entitled *Change Your Tastes* reviews the science behind our taste buds and why particular foods are more appealing than others. The section examines the element of pleasure in eating and how experiencing pleasure through food reinforces our consumption of those foods. Dr. Bacon also reviews the importance of genetics in our experience with taste, which helps to explain why some people can't stand bitter tastes, whereas others barely notice them. These two types of people represent the extremes in taste and are referred to as super-tasters and non-tasters, respectively. Super-tasters, for example, are likely to have a more restricted range of foods they find pleasurable to eat and are likely to reject certain types of plant-based foods due to their inherent bitterness. This means that how particular foods are prepared will matter so that they are enjoyable to eat. Food non-tasters are likely to have a less discriminatory palate allowing a wider variety of foods onto their plate; however, they may also be more prone to overeating. For non-tasters the recommendation is to pay closer attention to how foods taste, and to specifically include foods that particularly taste good. Beyond this particular genetic influence the section on Change Your Tastes reviews the evidence for why sugar is a powerful substance that many people seem to crave, how context and experience affect what we eat and what we enjoy eating, and whether or not particular foods can result in a food addiction.

As noted above, the HAES® approach was not developed to be a diet or a weight loss plan. The approach aims to help people shed the drive toward weight loss and learn to reconnect with themselves and their body so that they treat it in ways that promote their health. The idea is that when we engage in healthy behaviors we are likely to improve our overall health regardless of the shape and size our bodies are or what they become as a result of following the HAES® approach. Dr. Bacon suggests that when we let go of the cultural ideal of becoming and being thin we can learn to love our bodies for what they are capable of doing for us and will subsequently choose to direct our efforts to being sure our bodies are well taken care of rather than being sure it is a certain size.

What Is the Evidence that This Approach Is Effective?

Dr. Linda Bacon, founder of the HAES® approach intended to help people reframe their views on weight, health, and body size. She recognized that she developed this approach within a culture whose mantra was (and continues to be) if you are thin you are healthy, and if you are fat you are unhealthy and should do everything possible to become thin. Anything else is viewed as a path to disease and an early death. Dr. Bacon recognized that her approach went against what most health-care professionals and researchers espoused and continue to recommend. In her discussion of how she went about studying her approach, she noted that she wanted to be sure that she would not unfairly bias the results in favor of her approach. She stated that she recruited other researchers not only well-known in the areas of dieting and obesity but who also diverged from her opinion that weight loss was not the answer to improved health. She therefore reportedly recruited researchers who, if anything, would be skeptical of the HAES® approach and would work to ensure that there was not undue bias in favor of the approach. Dr. Bacon detailed the nature of this initial research project in terms of recruiting participants and how she secured funding for the project. Ultimately, this research team was able to recruit enough participants to divide them into two groups: one group worked through an early version of the HAES® approach as led by Dr. Bacon, and the other group worked with a registered dietician on the importance of starting and maintaining a diet. The results of the study, she reported, provided support for the HAES® approach.

Measures of how effective each leader was for their particular group (i.e., Dr. Bacon for the HAES® approach, and an experienced registered dietician for the diet group) were rated equally high suggesting that any differences found between the two groups were not due to the leaders themselves. Participants in the HAES® group were found to have moved away from dieting (restrictive eating) and toward a more intuitive eating style eating whatever foods they wanted when they were hungry and stopping when they were full. Although those in the diet group did show weight loss and improvements in their overall health, these results reportedly did not last. Those in the HAES® group were found to have lasting declines in bad cholesterol and blood pressure, reported significant increases in energy levels, and felt better about and in their bodies. The HAES® participants were also found to experience psychological benefits via increases in self-esteem and decreases in negative body image. In the diet group, these measures remained the same or got worse. Finally, the study revealed that nearly 50 percent of those who started in the diet group dropped out, whereas less than 8 percent in the HAES® group dropped out.

Dr. Bacon and her colleagues noted that what did not happen for either group in any meaningful way was weight loss. The HAES® group did not lose enough weight for it to be scientifically significant. The diet group did lose weight but then gained it all back—a finding consistent with other research on weight loss and diets. Those who participated in the HAES® group were found to have internalized the idea that the number on the scale was not as meaningful or important as how they felt not only in terms of liking themselves but also in terms of having improved health and energy. The authors concluded that the results dispelled the idea that exercising and eating healthier would lead to weight loss. Support for this conclusion has been found in some current research showing that weight loss, weight gain, or weight maintenance is far more complex than calories consumed versus calories burned.

Since the development of this approach and Dr. Bacon and colleagues' initial study of the HAES® approach, it has been studied by other researchers to determine if there truly are health benefits to the approach and what place, if any, it has in health care. A paper published in 2011 by Dr. Bacon and Lucy Aphramor examined the studies conducted by other scientists that looked at the HAES® approach in comparison to traditional dieting. The studies included in their article were randomized control trials (RTCs) which are currently the type that most researchers believe to be the most effective in determining whether one treatment or intervention is superior to another.

Since the HAES® approach is relatively new there were not many published RTCs; however, those that had been published seemed to show that the HAES® approach (or other approaches that refer to "size acceptance") was more effective and healthier in comparison to traditional dieting.

All six of the RCTs reviewed by Bacon and Aphramor showed that the HAES® approach reliably resulted in an improvement in health-related behaviors such as increased physical activity and reduced pathological eating patterns, and improvements in factors such as mood, self-esteem, and body image. Three of the four studies that measured health-related indicators such as blood pressure and blood lipids (fatty acids and cholesterol) reported statistically and clinically significant improvement. An additional factor the authors noted to be important was retention rate within the study. They note that among traditional weight loss programs drop-out is quite high and can result in yo-yo dieting, which has been shown to have significant negative health consequences. However, among the HAES®-type approaches retention was equal to or much higher than traditional weight loss programs. They concluded that in aggregate these studies show promise for size acceptance programs like the HAES® approach. The studies were found to have yielded positive results not only in terms of psychological well-being but also in terms of physical health. Bacon and Aphramor concluded that since size acceptance approaches were shown to outperform traditional weight loss programs and that people were more likely to stick with an approach like this compared to traditional weight loss or dieting, a strong case is being established for size acceptance approaches to be the go-to intervention in health-care fields. In an article published in 2014 in the *American Journal of Public Health*, author Andrea Bombak seems to have come to this conclusion as well.

Bombak noted that since the evidence has been mounting on the connection between obesity and myriad health risks, traditional approaches to eradicating obesity have failed. She reports that study after study examining weight-focused approaches have failed to produce effective results and suggests that a non-weight-centric approach should be taken when it comes to public health initiatives. She specifically names the HAES® approach as showing promise when it comes to implementing an effective public health prevention strategy.

Although much research is still needed to support the HAES® approach, the research conducted thus far suggests that it may be a viable alternative to traditional diet plans. As with any plan designed to address health concerns, it is always a good idea to consult with a licensed medical provider to ensure that any approach selected is safe given one's current health status.

WHAT ARE THE ONGOING CONCERNS ABOUT THIS APPROACH?

As noted in previous sections, the HAES® approach has been the focus of scientific study. This approach has been studied among premenopausal women, it has been combined with other forms of therapy to enhance overall acceptance of one's self, and it has been applied to clinical and educational settings. These and other studies suggest that this is a promising and appropriate approach to addressing health regardless of body size. But what about those who remain skeptical of the safety of HAES® for those who are obese and worry that this is just political-correctness gone too far? This section addresses these and other concerns about the HAES® approach.

Concerns about the HAES® approach include the idea that being fat is an automatic health risk that will end someone's life sooner than if they were not fat. Critics of the approach, therefore, suggest that it is irresponsible and dangerous to not actively encourage and work with overweight and obese people to lose weight. They are concerned that by saying weight has no bearing on health the result will be significant health problems months and maybe years later. For example, Dr. David Katz Director of the Prevention Research Center at Yale University was quoted as saying that while he agrees with the intent behind the approach that people should not be judged on their weight, he unequivocally states that weight is an indicator of health risk and that excess body fat is an identified risk factor for many major chronic diseases. Others who believe similarly encourage a distinction between thinking that weight should perhaps not be the most important factor when considering health and that it has no bearing on someone's health status at all.

Scientists Amanda Sainsbury and Phillipa Hay share the concerns of Dr. Katz and others. They contend that the research clearly shows that it is only a matter of time before all who are obese, including those who do not have metabolic syndrome, become seriously ill. They write that preventing weight gain as early as possible should be the goal of all individuals and health-care providers since once weight is put on it is more difficult to lose. They add that the longer excess weight is kept the more likely it is that there will be neurological and physiological changes making fat storage and ultimately weight gain much more efficient. Sainsbury and Hay acknowledge that very low calorie diets ultimately backfire by making people more hungry, which is the body's response to being under- or malnourished. Thus, these researchers state that they are in favor of healthy behaviors regardless of someone's body size as long as part of the focus is preventing weight gain or losing excess weight that has already been stored.

A common criticism of the HAES® approach is that it is a reflection of an all too politically correct society. Critics are concerned that the approach may send the message that you don't have to worry about your weight at all and that it is off limits for others to comment on it or be concerned about it. The end result, some believe, is that the HAES® approach may actually encourage people to stay unhealthy. Sainsbury and Hay indirectly address this by saying that the excessive concern our society has toward body size which has been accompanied by an overall increase in average body weight can lead to increasing mental health issues. They note that such a focus can lead to the increase that is seen in eating disorders and body dissatisfaction among a significant proportion of both males and females. Thus, being heavily focused on our own and others' body weight, shape, and size can have unintended and serious consequences suggesting that effective approaches to talking about and managing body-weight-related concerns are needed.

Regardless of one's support of or concern about this approach, researchers Tarra Penney and Sara Kirk suggest moving beyond ideology and focusing attention and resources on what truly improves the health of those who are experiencing stigma and health concerns. They also suggest that the HAES® approach does not have enough empirical support, at this point, to make it an approach that should inform public policy and clinical practice. In the chapters that follow some of the concerns raised by these and other researchers and practitioners will be addressed. For example, Chapter 7 explicitly examines the question of whether or not obese bodies can be healthy. Prior to addressing that controversy, Chapter 6 will focus on whether or not a focus on body shape and size will lead to overall well-being and happiness.

PART II

Controversies and Issues

CHAPTER 6

Body Image and Happiness: Should We Be Focused on Body Shape and Size?

The controversy over whether or not we should change our body shape and size by losing weight is a complex one. On the one hand, having a smaller body for women and a leaner, muscular body for men is currently deemed to be attractive and ideal in western cultures. Additionally, attractiveness is associated with socioeconomic and personal benefits that less attractive people are less likely to experience, and these benefits can lead to greater overall happiness. So, why not pursue dieting and weight-loss measures in order to be happier? Why not do everything we can to ensure that we are attractive as possible? The answer to this may be found in examining what role body image specifically plays in overall happiness and life satisfaction.

PROMISES OF WHAT WILL COME WITH THE IDEAL BODY SHAPE AND SIZE

Regardless of the time period being considered, the ideal body of the day is believed to come with certain promises. These promises are not always explicitly stated nor is there any kind of binding contract stating that if we achieve the ideal body then we are guaranteed these things. Nonetheless, when the ideal body is depicted there are advantages and benefits that allegedly accompany such a look. Achieving a particular body type, we are told, will lead to being a happier person, being more accepted and loved by others, being more successful, having a better sex life, overall being more attractive to the opposite sex, and being healthier.

In their eating disorder prevention program entitled *The Body Project: Promoting Body Acceptance and Preventing Eating Disorders,* authors Eric Stice and Katherine Presnell suggest that participants of the program dissect the current ideal body for females (the thin ideal) and suggest that participants answer questions such as "Where did this ideal come from?" "How is the thin ideal promoted to us?" and "How do messages about the thin ideal impact how you feel about yourself?" One of the final questions of this part of the program are "What does our culture tell us will happen if we are able to look like the thin ideal?" Stice and Presnell note that possible answers include many of the things listed earlier: acceptance, love, happiness, success, and wealth.

There is evidence to suggest that being attractive by current societal standards comes with certain advantages. Judith Langlois and colleagues reviewed hundreds of journal articles in an effort to determine if physical attractiveness is easily observed by others (rather than being "in the eye of the beholder"), and if those identified as attractive are treated differently than those who are not considered to be attractive. They concluded that attractiveness based on culture is something that is generally agreed upon. That is, most people in a particular society will agree on what and who is considered attractive. Research in this area indicates that attractive people (children and adults) are viewed more positively by others than those who are considered to be unattractive. This holds true regardless of whether or not the person is a friend or a stranger—your friends and family in addition to random strangers will judge you more positively if you are attractive than if you are not. The researchers also reported that it did not matter if the attractive person was male or female, or young or old—being attractive was beneficial regardless of sex or age. Attractive children and adults are more likely to be popular and adults more successful than their less attractive counterparts. Attractive children were found to be more well adjusted overall than unattractive children, and attractive compared to less attractive adults were found to have higher self-confidence and self-esteem, better mental health, and more dating experiences. Interestingly, the studies examined by Langlois and her colleagues on attractiveness and physical health revealed that there was no overall difference in physical health between those who are attractive and those who are not.

It is fair to conclude that being attractive may actually provide you with greater benefits than not being attractive would; however, what may not be accurate to conclude is that any one person would be guaranteed these and other benefits. Additionally, experiencing more success, more popularity, more wealth, more dating, and so on, will not likely look like what is promised via magazines, Hollywood, and the media in general. We will not become supermodels, make millions of dollars, or date the most eligible and attractive people. This is the promise that is made to the general public by popular media—"If you look like this, you can have what I have." This promise is what leads many of us to spend thousands of dollars over our lifetimes on beauty-related products designed to help us achieve a more attractive look. This promise is what leads human beings to spend billions of dollars world-wide on fitness and beauty-related products so we can finally achieve the ideal look and be granted the benefits we are promised.

THE BILLION-DOLLAR BEAUTY INDUSTRY

Attractiveness is unique to each culture and each era. What is attractive now in the United States was not attractive in this country several decades ago, and would not be considered attractive by other contemporary cultures. As discussed in Chapter 1, history shows us that no matter what the standard people are willing to sacrifice their bodies and their wallets in order to more closely approximate the current ideal. What has changed in the past few decades is the staggering amount of money people are willing to spend to get there. Globally, people purchase gym memberships and individual sessions with personal trainers, cosmetics designed to enhance or cover up what is already there, surgery to do the same, and colognes and perfumes to ensure that we smell good to potential dating partners. The total amount spent each year can be measured in the hundreds of billions of dollars.

In 2003, an article in *The Economist* reported that human beings across the globe are willing to spend over $160 billion a year to achieve whatever look is deemed attractive by the society in which they live. It is likely that that number is closer to if not over $200 billion at the time of the writing of this book. According to Statista.com, the United States spent over $40 billion in 2002 on cosmetics alone and that number was projected to be over $62 billion in 2016. This site also reported that the amount spent on cosmetic surgery in the United States is also measured in the billions of dollars. In 2015 people in the United States spent over $8 billion on plastic surgery. The weight-loss market specifically was measured at over $60 billion dollars in 2013 and is project to exceed $65 billion as of 2016.

We are spending billions of dollars to temporarily alter our perceived attractiveness by applying perfumes and cosmetics, and by engaging in some kind of weight-loss endeavor with the hopes of losing the weight for good. Some of us are also looking for something more permanent and are willing to spend hundreds or thousands of dollars on elective surgical procedures, again with the hopes of improving our attractiveness. Ultimately, the expectation is not only that our looks will improve but that our lives will improve also. As noted in the previous section, there is some evidence to suggest that being more attractive does have benefits that may include happiness.

One study examining attractiveness or beauty and happiness indicates that these two concepts seem go hand in hand. The researchers reported that the more attractive someone is the more resources and benefits (e.g., popularity, income) they enjoy, and this leads to greater overall happiness. But is there a caveat to the relationship between attractiveness and happiness? That is, why might someone who is objectively attractive be unhappy even if they are receiving the benefits that come with attractiveness? Another line of research offers an answer to this question.

ARE PEOPLE WITH BETTER BODIES HAPPIER?

The question of what contributes to someone's overall happiness has been debated for millennia. As with most things in life, the answer is not simple. Genetics in addition to determining eye color, height, and what sex we are also influences our overall happiness. However, researchers have found that things that are within our control like staying physically active, giving back to one's community, and having solid relationships play a significant role in our overall happiness. But what about how we look? Does our appearance have direct bearing on our overall happiness? As noted in the previous section, being objectively attractive carries with it certain benefits. More attractive people are afforded more and better employment opportunities; they often have a wider range of dating partners from whom to pick, and attractive people are judged more favorably than those who are less attractive. So, does this mean that attractive people are also happier than less attractive people?

A study conducted as part of the *Discussion Paper Series* for the Institute for the Study of Labor (IZA) in Bonn, Germany, examined attractiveness and degree of attractiveness among males and females. They examined data collected in the United States, Canada, the United Kingdom, and Germany. These researchers relied on data that assessed attractiveness based on others' perceptions of attractiveness rather than peoples' opinions about their own attractiveness. Given the fact that attractiveness has consistently been linked to a variety of things that are often associated with being happy, it is not surprising that these researchers found that attractiveness or beauty is connected to overall happiness for both men and women, and that there is little difference between the two sexes.

The researchers noted, however, that the connection between these two constructs is explained primarily in indirect ways. That is, attractiveness affords greater opportunities for dating, job choices, and income which in turn can contribute to peoples' overall happiness. What was surprising, however, is that after examining the data collected across four countries there seems to be a significant direct (rather than indirect) effect on happiness for women. For women, if things like income, dating possibilities, and other factors often connected with happiness are ignored, being attractive on its own predicted their level of happiness.

Based on these findings objectively attractive people are happier than less attractive people. But what if we do not view *ourselves* as attractive? We may be perceived as being attractive by others, but what if we don't view ourselves so favorably? One way in which people judge themselves and their overall attractiveness is in terms of the size and shape of their bodies. How one feels about one's body is usually referred to as body image. Having a positive body image means that one view's one's body favorably (i.e., they like their body), whereas having a negative body image means that one views one's body less favorably (i.e., they don't like their body).

Rachel Stokes and Christina Frederick-Recascino set out to determine if women's body image is connected to happiness. They predicted that when women felt better about their bodies (i.e., the have a positive body image) they would be happier. The researchers used a measure of body esteem which they noted is a term often used interchangeably with body image. This particular measure included three elements of body image or body esteem, which were sexual attractiveness, weight concern, and physical condition. The idea is that body esteem is not a single construct or idea but a complex idea made up of at least these three components. The sexual attractiveness element refers to how attractive you think you are to other people—specifically those who might have a sexual interest in you. These second facet, weight concern, measured how someone feels about the parts of their body that might change through diet and exercise. The final factor, physical condition, refers to what your body is capable of—that is how much stamina you have, how agile you are, how strong you are, and so on. The results of their study supported their prediction.

Stokes and Frederick-Recascino found that each of the three elements of body esteem (i.e., one's perception of one's sexual attractiveness, weight concern, and physical condition) were related to one's overall happiness. It is important to clarify that this research is not identifying how other people feel about someone else, this study measured how people feel about themselves in terms of their bodies and whether or not this was in any way related to happiness. These researchers demonstrated that the more positive someone's body image or the higher their body esteem the happier they would be, and the lower their body image or body esteem the less happy they would be. The authors conclude that while this is an important finding, their study does not provide any information about cause and effect. Research thus far has not been able to answer the question as to whether or not having a higher body image causes happiness or if being happy causes someone to have a higher body image. Regardless, the connection between the two suggests that when considering what makes people happy, it is possible that body image is part of that equation.

A more recent study conducted by researchers associated with You-Beauty.com also examined the connection between body image and happiness. In their study, the YouBeauty.com Body Image Survey (YBIS), the researchers agreed with Stokes and Frederick-Recascino and noted that body image is not a simple construct, and that it includes multiple dimensions that can make it challenging to fully understand and study. They identified one such element as body appreciation which is defined as being able to think and feel positively about one's body regardless of how it looks. Body appreciation therefore involves a degree of respect for one's body that ignores societal expectations of the ideal body. Individuals with high body appreciation give their body what it needs and accept it as it is.

The results of the YBIS indicated that body appreciation is positively correlated with happiness—meaning that the higher a woman's body appreciation the higher her reported level of happiness and vice versa. The researchers reported that their findings are consistent with the results of myriad other studies and recommended that professionals help women live happier and more fulfilling lives and work with their clients to improve body appreciation by helping them focus more on how their body works rather than on how it looks. By doing so, they will be able to develop a greater appreciation and respect for their body.

While the overall conclusion that feeling good about one's body is linked to greater overall happiness was based on their survey of many women, the authors of the YBIS study noted that nearly 90 percent of the women in their study reported feeling dissatisfied with their weight and most wanted to lose weight. They noted that this finding, too, was consistent with what other researchers have found. Thus, while the good news is that appreciating one's body in terms of how it functions means we are more likely to be happy, most women are focused on how their bodies look and are not happy with what they see. Consequently, women are more likely than their body appreciating counterparts to be less happy overall.

WOULD YOU REALLY BE HAPPIER IF YOU LOOKED BETTER?

Would you really be happier if you looked better? This is the title of an article published in 2016 and examines the effect of something called the *focusing illusion*. The authors of this article applied the focusing illusion to how people perceive their bodies and their overall degree of happiness. Initially, the focusing illusion was applied to whether or not living in a particular geographical location would make people happier.

In their 1998 article on whether or not living in California will make people happier, researchers David Schkade and Daniel Kahneman first used the term focusing illusion. They coined this term to describe the phenomenon whereby people overestimate the impact of a single event or experience on their overall happiness. They noted that a study published in 1978 by Brickman, Coates, and Janoff-Bulman revealed the surprising and perhaps even shocking finding that when comparing lottery winners to paraplegics on overall life satisfaction there was no difference. This means that winning the lottery or not having the ability to use all of one's limbs did not dictate how happy someone was. For most people this is likely counterintuitive. Some readers may even find that difficult to believe. If we are able-bodied and think about what it might be like to lose the functioning of our arms and/or our legs we imagine that our lives will be irreparably changed for the worse, whereas the opposite would be true of winning a large sum of money. This is precisely what the focusing illusion helps to explain. When we focus on one thing or place more importance on that one thing in terms of our overall happiness, we have the tendency to overestimate the degree to which it will actually affect our happiness. Research in the area of happiness supports this finding. In fact, one of the most well-known researchers in the area of happiness, Daniel Gilbert, has extensively studied what contributes to our overall happiness and our individual understanding of what makes us happy.

Gilbert and his colleagues have examined a concept known as *affective forecasting,* which refers to our ability to predict how long we will be emotionally impacted by a particular event. For example, these researchers wondered what people's predictions would be about how long they would feel badly about the breakup of a romantic relationship or how badly or happy they would feel after they were denied or received a promotion. Overall, they found that no matter the event or situation that evoked a particular emotional response participants consistently overestimated how long they would continue to feel the way they did. It did not matter if the event was a positive event (e.g., received a promotion) or a negative one (e.g., end of a romantic relationship). These findings taken along with the work related to the focusing illusion helps to explain why large changes in our lives such as winning the lottery or becoming a paraplegic will impact our lives as we might expect but it will only do so temporarily. Eventually we adapt to our new circumstances and focus on other things in our lives that also affect happiness such as work, family, friends, and so on. Thus, our overall happiness might suffer or improve when significant events occur, but we will, after a relatively short period of time, return to a level of happiness that is similar to where we were to begin with.

These findings have direct implications for the beauty industry and weight loss in particular. Weight loss and body transformation programs and products promise that users' lives will be vastly improved if only they change the way they look. Schkade and Kahneman predicted that it is relatively easy to exploit the effect of the focusing illusion by promising dramatic changes or results with a seemingly minor change: "just take this" or "just do this" and your life will be dramatically better. Gilbert and colleagues' work would further predict that such promises will come true for a short period of time and may therefore feel like our lives have dramatically changed and will stay that way. However, the degree to which someone was happy or unhappy prior to using a weight loss product or program is where they will return to after a relatively brief period of time. Thus, the actual customers one might see in a commercial advertising a weight-loss product or program who appear to be happy about their transformation are likely quite happy at that time. However, if one could see their overall happiness weeks or months later, the research would predict these same people would not likely to be as happy as they were immediately following their weight loss.

Lukasz Kaczmarek and colleagues applied the focusing illusion concept to body image and life satisfaction. They noted that not all areas of one's life are subject to the effects of the focusing illusion but that research shows important areas such as income, dating, marriage, and health are. They further noted that understanding which areas in people lives they might overestimate in terms of its effect on life satisfaction are important to identify. Thus, these researchers were interested in determining if a focus on body satisfaction or body image would be subject to the focusing illusion effect. Their results suggested that it is. When people are focused on their overall satisfaction with their body, they tend to overestimate how much this impacted their happiness. Therefore, if someone is dissatisfied with their body they are likely to assume that if they change their body (e.g., lose weight) then they will be happier and their lives will be much improved. If they continue to focus solely on this one aspect of who they are, the focusing illusion suggests that they will not be as happy as they imagine they would be once the newness of losing weight has worn off.

Research show us that those who are attractive have more figurative doors open to them in terms of friendships, dating, employment, and ultimately income. It is not surprising then that attractiveness has been connected with degree of happiness. This research, however, often measures attractiveness in terms of other people's perceptions of beauty. Thus, if someone else finds you attractive, they are more likely to bestow upon you the benefits discussed in the beginning of this chapter. However, when one considers attractiveness in terms of how one feels about one's self, research shows that the more positively one feels about themselves the happier they are. Some of this research has shown that when women focus their attention to how their body functions rather than how it looks they are more likely to report being happier. The caveat to all this is found in the focusing illusion, which reminds us that if being attractive—which for many people means losing weight or staying thin—is one's sole focus for happiness then once their desired appearance is achieved they are likely to find that they are not as happy as they predicted they would be.

CHAPTER 7

Can Overweight or Obese Bodies Really Be Healthy?

The average body size of citizens of the United States has been on the rise for the past several decades. What this has meant is that more and more people are classified as overweight or obese (as measured by BMI—see Chapter 2 for a discussion of BMI). The increasing numbers in these classifications is due in part to the increase in average body size, but also due to changing thresholds for what constitutes an overweight or obese body. Regardless of what the average weight of a population is or how that is measured, one question that has been fairly controversial is whether or not someone can be overweight or obese and be healthy. Culturally we tend to equate thinness with health, and fatness with lack of health. There are a multitude of studies linking obesity to various diseases and illnesses; however, critics of this body of research suggest that since these studies are correlational in nature it is inappropriate to conclude that being fat causes these health problems. Critics also note that fat people are rarely depicted in various forms of media as engaging in healthy activities (e.g., exercise) and enjoying it or being happy. They contend that this kind of bias further fuels the notion that people who are overweight or obese are unhealthy and unhappy, and the only viable solution being to lose weight.

This section will summarize some of the research on the medical issues associated with overweight and obesity, and discuss what many health-care providers and policy makers have concluded based on these findings. Also examined will be a growing body of research looking at whether or not weight loss can be maintained long term and whether or not it produces the health benefits many believe weight loss should. Finally, newly published longevity studies will be presented suggesting that people with a body size larger than many would have predicted live longer than their thinner and more overweight counterparts.

DISEASES LINKED TO OBESITY

In 2013 obesity was classified as a disease by the American Medical Association (AMA). This was due in part to the fact that so many other diseases have been connected to obesity that the AMA and others determined that obesity was not merely a risk factor for these diseases but was a serious problem in and of itself. Given the AMA's decision to classify obesity as a disease it is not surprising that efforts of various companies, governmental agencies, and health-care providers have turned toward helping people lose weight so they are no longer overweight or obese. The idea is to reduce someone's weight so they are no longer obese and are therefore no longer unhealthy. Despite the strong and clear stand of the AMA, critics of this decision argue that not all people who are obese are unhealthy. Some counter this observation with the idea that it is merely a matter of time before a now healthy obese person becomes unhealthy. This begs the question: Are overweight and obese people automatically unhealthy? This section will take a look at some of the diseases that are linked to being overweight or obese, and will be followed by a separate section examining why the connection between obesity and health may not be as clear as it would seem.

Diabetes

Diabetes, specifically type 2 diabetes mellitus, has been linked to obesity for many years. Evidence has shown that as BMI increases so does the risk for developing type 2 diabetes. In studies of men and women, the risk for developing type 2 diabetes increases 2 to 5 times, respectively, with a BMI in the overweight category (i.e., BMI of 25) and continues to exponentially increase with a BMI of 30 and again at a BMI of 35. For men with a BMI over 35 the risk is 42 times greater than someone with a BMI of 21 or less, and for women the risk is 93 times greater.

The medical explanation for why obesity should have such a dramatic impact on whether or not someone develops type 2 diabetes involves understanding how body fat influences the metabolism of glucose. Glucose refers to blood sugar; blood sugar or glucose levels are affected by the foods we eat. Insulin is a hormone that helps the body to metabolize glucose and helps to regulate glucose levels so they do not get too high (hyperglycemia) or too low (hypoglycemia). In short, insulin allows the body's cells to use sugar for energy and helps store excess sugar for later use if needed. Diabetes occurs when insulin function is compromised.

An individual with type 1 diabetes has a body that cannot make insulin and therefore they require regular insulin injections so their body can adequately process glucose. Without the injections someone with type 1 diabetes would become hyperglycemic (too much blood sugar because there is not enough insulin to help the body use the blood sugar). Results of hyperglycemia include damage to the nerves, kidneys, blood vessels in the eyes, and damage to the heart and blood vessels which can increase the risk of heart attack or stroke. Individuals with type 2 diabetes are able to produce insulin however their bodies are unable to adequately use the insulin which means they too are at risk for hyperglycemia. Changing one's diet and introducing or increasing exercise are common treatments for type 2 diabetes; however, the longer someone has this particular type of diabetes the greater the chances they will need insulin treatments to regulate their glucose levels.

The link between obesity and processing blood sugar involves, in part, the degree of upper body fat someone has. Studies have shown that the more upper body fat someone has the more likely their body will be resistant to insulin. In other words, the more fat someone carries in their upper body (i.e., waist up) the more likely it is that their body will not be able to use the insulin it produces. Other studies have shown that depending on the location of fat deposits in the body, the body is more or less responsive to hormones responsible for adequately processing or breaking down body fat. Related to this issue is the release of free fatty acids which have been linked to insulin resistance and inflammation. The compromised responsiveness to the hormones used to break down body fat results in an increase in free fatty acids present in one's system which in turn hinders the adequate functioning of insulin.

The finding that upper body fat is linked to problems adequately processing blood sugar has led to the connection between diabetes and obesity.

Cardiovascular Disease

Cardiovascular disease refers generally to problems with the heart and blood vessels. We can be born with a condition that can cause cardiovascular disease; however, most causes stem from factors that are within our control, including smoking, what we eat, and how much exercise we get. Being overweight or obese has also been identified as a risk factor. This risk factor is explained in terms of the growth of one's body such that as the body grows more skin is present on the body which is accompanied by an increase in fat and muscle mass. This leads to an increase in overall blood volume; larger bodies have more blood. With more blood comes an increased demand on the heart and for some people this can lead to hypertension or a consistent elevation in blood pressure as well as an enlargement in the left ventricle of the heart which is the heart's primary pumping chamber. This type of change in one's body can lead to changes in the structure of the heart as well as how effectively it works. The results can include a weakened heart or loss of elasticity which can further lead to inadequate blood supply to the heart, inadequate blood supply to the body, or an abnormal heart beat.

Although the increased risk for cardiovascular disease is not as dramatic as that found between obesity and diabetes, the risk of cardiovascular problems, specifically coronary heart disease, increases as BMI increases. One study reported that obese men and women younger than 50 years old were 2 times and just under 2.5 times greater risk, respectively, for coronary heart disease.

Cancer

Although the word cancer conjures fear in a lot of people, the reality is that cancer simply refers to abnormal cell growth. The fear of cancer, of course, comes with the devastating effects this abnormal cell growth can cause. And because some cancers are untreatable altogether or cannot be cured if identified too late, the fear of cancer involves the possibility of dying.

The National Cancer Institute (NCI) notes that much of the data connecting cancer to obesity was collected by looking at specific cohorts of people (i.e., studying groups people who are the same in all ways but one—smokers and nonsmokers), and observational studies which involve simply measuring certain things about people such as whether or not they have cancer, what their BMI is, what their eating habits are like, and so on. Cohort studies can provide a clearer but not definitive picture of what may be a strong risk factor for a particular disease by starting with people who don't have the disease, following them over time and seeing which group (e.g., smokers or nonsmokers) has more incidences of the disease. Observational studies do not collect data in this way, rather they simply observe who has and who does not have the disease right now and what characteristics they may or may not have in common.

Although both types of research have shortcomings, the data in aggregate show a strong connection between obesity and several types of cancer which include, but is not limited to, endometrial cancer, liver cancer, kidney cancer, colorectal cancer, breast cancer, ovarian cancer, and thyroid cancer. The NCI notes that there may be several factors contributing to why those who are obese have higher rates of cancer which can include chronic low-level inflammation, fat tissue, and higher levels of insulin.

Inflammation in the body has been linked to various diseases including cancer. If inflammation is not reduced or eliminated, the result can be changes to an individual's DNA, which can then contribute to the development of cancer. Having a certain amount of fatty tissue stored in the body, particularly for women, has health benefits; however, having higher amounts can result in the overproduction of the hormone estrogen, which is linked to certain types of cancer (e.g., breast cancer, endometrial cancer). Fat cells can also affect the rate of cell growth which when abnormal is the very definition of cancer. Finally, and as discussed in the section on diabetes, individuals who are obese show greater levels of insulin which, in addition to being implicated in the development of type 2 diabetes, has also been linked to the development of cancers, such as colon cancer, kidney cancer, prostate cancer, and endometrial cancer.

In addition to studying the connection between cancer and obesity, the NCI states that avoiding weight gain during adulthood may decrease one's risk for developing cancer in the first place. They note, however, that research looking at weight loss and a reduced risk of cancer is not quite as strong with the exception of weight loss due to bariatric surgery. As indicated in the context of obesity and rates of cancer, the NCI indicates that definitive conclusions cannot be drawn from these findings given the type of research conducted and other factors (e.g., method used to lose weight) that may help to explain the findings.

Sleep Apnea and Other Sleep-Related Breathing Problems

Researchers indicate that the respiratory system can be compromised due to an increase in body fat. They indicate that the working of the diaphragm and chest can be altered by increased body fat and that this interference is exacerbated when an obese individual lies on their back. The lungs are not able to inflate fully which in turn can lead to hypoxia (i.e., not enough oxygen circulating in the system) and hypercapnia (i.e., too much carbon dioxide which occurs when respiration is inadequate). The result of this process is that sleep is compromised by restlessness and consistent waking during sleep.

Sleep apnea is a sleep disorder that involves the cessation of breathing during sleep. There are two types of sleep apnea: obstructive sleep apnea and central sleep apnea. Of the two types, obstructive sleep apnea is the most common. This type occurs when the airway is blocked as a result of soft tissue in the back of the throat collapsing and obstructing the airway. Central sleep apnea has to do with the brain's inability to signal the body to breathe as it normally would.

There is some degree of normal disruption in the ratio of oxygen and carbon dioxide in the respiratory system during rapid eye movement (REM) sleep. Episodes of apnea (i.e., cessation of breathing) can occur among all sleepers regardless of body size but is reportedly more pronounced among those who are obese. Although lack of sleep in and of itself can result in low energy and feeling poorly overall, chronic lack of sleep can increase the risk for cardiac problems and cerebral problems such as stroke.

Nonalcoholic Fatty Liver Disease

Fatty liver disease refers to excess fat accumulated in the liver and is usually associated with overconsumption of alcohol. By contrast, nonalcoholic fatty liver disease (NAFLD) is the same in that there is a buildup of fat in the liver, but it is not caused by overconsumption of alcohol. According to the American Liver Foundation (ALF), fat is considered to be excessive when more than 5–10 percent of the liver's weight is from fat. At this point, the liver is considered diseased and is called fatty liver or steatosis. The AFD indicates that approximately 25 percent of people in the United States can be diagnosed with NAFLD and higher rates are associated with a higher BMI. In nonobese people, around 15 percent may have NAFLD whereas in the highest range of obesity the rate can be as high as 85 percent.

According to the ALF, non-alcoholic fatty liver disease is found predominantly in those who are overweight or obese. They also note that having diabetes is a risk factor for developing this disease as is not eating well. Interestingly, the ALF also reports that losing weight in a short period of time may also be a risk factor in developing NAFLD. Finally, the ALF states that NAFLD can develop in people who do not have any of the identified risk factors. One their website, the ALF provides a case example of a marathon runner who was diagnosed with NAFLD despite his being a health nut.

A study conducted in 2010 examined obesity and NAFLD, which included looking at medical markers associated with metabolic health such as insulin resistance, inflammation, fatty acid metabolism, and so on, which may contribute to the development of NAFLD. They found that although these issues are associated with obesity as many as 30 percent of those who are obese are considered to be metabolically normal.

Overall the researchers concluded that it is not clear whether NAFLD is a result of metabolic problems, or if the presence of NFALD itself leads to the development of metabolic problems. Thus, although the connection between obesity and NAFLD exists, the nature of the connection seems to be unclear.

Osteoarthritis

Osteoarthritis (OA) refers to a form of joint disease that according to the Arthritis Foundation (AF) is the most common chronic problem found in people's joints. OA is also referred to as "wear and tear" arthritis since it was once believed to be the result of repeated use of the joints. Those dealing with OA often experience stiffness after not moving for a period of time (e.g., sleeping, sitting) or overusing the joints, and pain. OA often affects the hips, knees, fingers, feet, and lower back and those experiencing this form of arthritis may notice cracking or grinding in the joints, difficult moving a joint or limited range of motion, and pain that increase with activity or by the end of one's day. OA itself can affect ones' quality of life and has the possibility of leading to someone becoming more sedentary. This can, in turn, lead to the development of more serious conditions such as diabetes or heart disease.

The AF notes that there is no single cause of OA and it is not merely a result of chronic wear and tear. They note that certain genetic traits can predispose someone to developing OA as young as one's early 20s. Injuring or overusing a joint can also lead to OA, a cause which can be found among many athletes. Repetitive movement of a joint or an injury to the joint can damage tendons and ligaments, and ultimately lead to the breakdown of the cartilage that exists between the bones of the joint. Finally, the AF identifies weight as a contributing factor to the development of OA. They note that the more weight one carries the more pressure is put on various joints including the hips and knees. Being overweight for many years can accelerate the degeneration of cartilage resulting in OA and its accompanying symptoms. There may also be a link between obesity and OA in the hands as research has connected chemicals associated with inflammation (which is linked to excess fat) and damage to the joints.

The research examining obesity and the diseases discussed earlier paints a fairly grim picture. There is a great deal of evidence linking obesity with these diseases which implies that obesity is the reason, or an important reason, for the development of these disorders. It is clear, however, that obesity cannot be the sole factor in the development of these diseases since research on each one has noted that these diseases are also diagnosed independent of obesity. The research that does connect obesity with these diseases has been met with strong criticism with regard to the conclusion that obesity causes these diseases to develop. The next section examines why critics call into question this cause-and-effect link.

WHY IS THIS RESEARCH IN QUESTION?

Generally speaking, when people consider the health of someone who is obese, there is often an automatic assumption that the person is already unhealthy. If they are not, then the assumption is that it is only a matter of time before they develop a debilitating disease. Either way, the extrapolation is that obese people will be sicker and are likely to die sooner than their normal weight counterparts unless they do something about it—which usually means weight loss. Recent research, however, has shed some light on whether or not obesity alone (as measured by BMI) is an adequate measure of someone's overall health or risk of premature death. This section will examine some of the research indicating that other methods need to be used to measure disease risk or risk of early death. Additional research will be summarized suggesting that individuals who are obese can, in fact, be healthy.

Those who write about obesity and challenge the firmly held notions about what obesity means to an individual as well as society at large acknowledge that obesity has been linked to numerous health concerns (e.g., heart disease, some forms of cancer, sleep problems) as well as an earlier death. What they question, however, is whether it is obesity that is the cause of these issues or if obesity is simply the most obvious explanation. Two researchers, Rexford Ahima and Mitchell Lazar, are among those who offer a contrasting view of how obesity ought to be thought about and approached in terms of health—they specifically challenge the veracity of using BMI as a measure of health risk. They summarize recent findings among researchers who have studied obesity and subsequently found that obesity may not be linked to as many problems as initially believed. They indicate that while using BMI allows for classification of individuals based on weight it is not an adequate measure for determining the overall health of an individual.

Ahima and Lazar note that BMI is incapable of measuring elements of the body and its composition that are more likely to accurately reflect the health of an individual. They suggest that in order to determine a person's degree of health it is important to know how much body fat the person has in addition to the ratio of muscle to fat. Similarly, Marjorie Bastien and her colleagues reached a similar conclusion in their examination of how obesity contributes to cardiovascular disease. They indicated that it is not so much the amount of fat an individual has that may increase their risk of cardiovascular disease rather it is the quality of the fat and how the fat functions that matters more.

With regard to body fat these researchers indicate that it is critical to understand fat content (i.e., type of fat) and where the fat is located in the body. Visceral fat (i.e., intra-abdominal fat), for example, is fat that is stored deep in the body in the abdominal area, whereas subcutaneous fat is stored just below the skin's surface. Either type of fat can result in an individual's stomach area being large and is often referred to as belly fat. More importantly, however, is that visceral fat specifically surrounds vital internal organs and changes how they function. This type of fat releases its own hormones and other substances that are known to cause inflammation. As such, visceral fat has been associated with some of the same diseases and health issues as obesity such as heart disease, cancer, stroke, diabetes, and arthritis. Although visceral fat is most obvious in those who are obese, this same type of fat can be found in those who are normal weight. Regardless of body size, having too much visceral fat is implicated in what is known as *metabolic syndrome*.

Metabolic syndrome involves a constellation of factors that put someone at greater risk for developing heart disease, diabetes, stroke, and other health problems. Having several of these factors indicates that someone likely has metabolic syndrome. These factors include a large waistline, which is indicative of a significant amount of visceral fat, high levels of a type of fat found in the blood stream called triglycerides, having a low level of the good (HDL) cholesterol, which in adequate levels helps to clear out cholesterol from the arteries, high blood pressure, and having a blood sugar level that is too high. While metabolic syndrome is linked to a number of serious health problems, studies examining the health of individuals with a variety of body sizes indicate that equating metabolic syndrome with obesity is erroneous.

Researchers Roger Unger and Phillipp Scherer out of the University of Texas Southwestern Medical Center at Dallas found that obese bodies that store fat subcutaneously (instead of viscerally) may keep toxins, which are stored in fat, away from vital organs. This has the effect of improved cardiovascular and metabolic health. These researchers also found that in addition to where the fat was stored the structure of the fat cells mattered in terms of degree of inflammation in the body. They noted that groupings of fat cells that were smaller, had blood vessels (as opposed to fat cells without blood vessels), and did not have an excessive amount of fibrous connective tissue (often associated with scarring) were found to be healthier and are referred to as healthy fat pads. They stated that when a grouping or pad of this type of healthy fat cells expands there is a greater chance that there will be less inflammation which in turn may be protective against insulin resistance. The growth of healthy fat pads is largely genetically determined and has been found to a greater degree among females compared to males.

In another study examining the relationship between inflammation, obesity, and diabetes, Vivian Luft and her colleagues found that although being obese was strongly tied to diabetes they also found that when taking into account a particular protein and various indicators of inflammation the risk of diabetes was cut by more than half. This meant that obesity alone was not the cause of diabetes. In fact, these authors stated that not only does inflammation predict the onset of diabetes it also predicts weight gain suggesting that it may be that inflammation is the causal mechanism of diabetes as well as obesity.

The research in the area of metabolic syndrome suggests that while it can be connected to those who are obese it can also be connected to those who are not obese. As such, these researchers suggest that looking at weight or BMI alone in an effort to predict or treat disease linked to obesity is not sufficient. They suggest that measures designed to better capture what truly makes up the metabolic syndrome will be more effective at predicting health risk.

Is Long-Term Weight Loss Truly Possible?

Perhaps no controversy related to body size is more volatile than whether or not weight loss is even possible. It is likely that most if not all people one may ask would say "Yes, weight loss is possible." They may point to their own weight loss or the weight loss of someone they know. The crux of this controversy is whether or not the weight lost is kept off for a meaningful length of time. Again, most people would say that their own weight loss or the weight loss of someone they know was sustained for quite a while. But how does one define long-term weight loss? Weight kept off for one year? Two years? More? This section will examine how long-term weight loss is defined. The section will also look at studies conducted to determine if long-term weight loss is possible as well as meta-analytic studies designed to draw conclusions based on the findings of a more than one study that asked the same (or a very similar) question.

The general positon that many people take about weight loss is that it is either relatively easy to accomplish or very difficult to do. Scientific articles regularly note that how much one weighs has multiple determinants.

That is, there is no signal thing that causes someone to be overweight or obese, thin, or normal weight. Research and medical professionals point to factors that include broad categories such as genetics, the environment, and psychosocial factors. This constellation of possible causes suggests that manipulating one's weight is likely not as easy as it might seem. Despite this, the second and seemingly contradictory positon about weight and weight loss is that manipulating weight is as simple as calories in and calories out. That is, if you burn more calories than you consume, then you will lose weight. This approach, then, presumes that weight loss, weight gain, or weight maintenance is entirely within the control of the individual. As such, if someone is not their ideal weight then responsibility for that rests squarely on their shoulders and it is their fault.

There are numerous studies indicating not only that weight loss is possible but that it can be maintained long term. A discussion of some of that research is next followed by research concluding that long-term weight loss is not possible.

Long-Term Weight Loss Is Possible

For decades since concern about obesity has made it to the public's awareness the prevailing solution for the obesity problem—which now is referred to as the obesity epidemic—is weight loss. Obesity has for so long been believed to be a problem in and of itself (and the American Medical Association declared obesity to be a disease in 2013) that the focus has historically been on making someone who is obese no longer obese. The only way to do that is to lose weight.

Researchers in a multitude of different fields including psychology, medicine, public health, and nutrition have attempted to figure out the best way to lose weight, to help people want to lose weight, and to help those who want to lose weight but who are struggling to sustain a weight loss program. These efforts have resulted in a fairly large body of literature suggesting that weight loss is not only possible it can be maintained.

In order to determine whether or not weight loss is really being maintained by those attempting to lose weight, it is important to clearly define what constitutes meaningful weight loss, and how long someone has to keep the weight off in order to say that they have maintained that weight loss. In 2001 researchers Rena Wing and James Hill recognized the lack of uniformity with respect to both meaningful weight loss and weight loss maintenance. They suggested a reasonable definition of weight loss maintenance would include someone having lost at least 10 percent of their overall body weight and that they maintained that loss for at least one year.

The one-year mark is often used to define not only weight loss maintenance but also long-term weight loss.

In their efforts to define and describe successful weight loss maintenance, this research team focused on the National Weight Control Registry (NWCR), which was founded in 1994. According to their website, at
the time of this writing the NWCR tracks over 10,000 adults 80 percent
of whom identify as female and 20 percent of whom identify as male. The
website also indicates that members of this group have lost an average of
66 pounds, which they have kept off for five and a half years. This was the
same amount of weight and length of time reported in their 2001 study. As
such, findings as promising as this led Wing and Hill to determine what
members of this group had in common so they could identify behaviors
that might prove successful for others to adopt. Thus, it was their intent to
study successful weight loss maintainers only (i.e., those who lost at least
10 percent of overall body weight and kept it off for at least one year).

Wing and Hill allow entry into the NWCR if adult applicants have lost
at least 30 pounds and kept that weight off for one year. Registry members complete a series of questionnaires designed to measure weight loss
efforts, weight maintenance behaviors, weight history, and so on. Similar
questionnaires are completed again annually. In their 2001 report, Wing
and Hill noted that approximately 90 percent of registry members had
previously tried and failed to lose weight adding that the only difference
now seemed to be that members were more strict with their dieting and
included exercise more prominently in their weight loss efforts. To that
end, Wing and Hill noted that most members did modify both their food
intake and physical activity rather than relying on changes to diet alone.
With respect to changes in food intake, registry members reported that
they tend to restrict certain types of food consumed, restrict the overall
amount of food consumed, and count calories. There was a mixture among
both sexes regarding whether or not they made these changes on their own
or if they followed a weight loss program of some kind.

In a follow-up article in 2005, Wing and Phelan concluded that based
on their research there are six things adults can do in order to achieve
long-term weight loss (i.e., losing at least 10% of one's body weight and
keeping it off for at least one year). The first two strategies involved diet
and exercise and are: ensuring that you are engaged in physical activity at
a high level, and eating foods that have low fat and eating fewer calories.
They also noted that it is important for adults to eat breakfast and establish an overall pattern of eating that is consistent. They also recommend
monitoring one's weight on a regular basis, and noticing slips (e.g., eating higher fat foods, not exercising, not weighing one's self) as soon as

possible so that they do not take hold thereby establishing a new pattern of behavior.

A number of scientists have examined the research as a whole on weight loss maintenance. They identified numerous studies that specifically looked at weight loss and whether or not that weight loss could be maintained. Their conclusions are based on looking at the findings of these studies in aggregate. Two articles published in 2005 and written by independent groups examined weight loss efforts and the degree to which these efforts were sustainable and meaningful in a setting outside of a research study.

Curioni and Lourenço examined studies comparing the effectiveness of making changes to food intake and physical activity compared to only changing food intake. They wanted to know what the research said about the effectiveness of diet plus exercise compared to diet alone when it comes to weight loss. They concluded that those who used diet and exercise to try to lose weight were more effective in their weight loss efforts that those who used dieting alone. Those who used diet and exercise lost more weight compared to those who used diet alone. Moreover, those who used the combined approach were more effective in keeping some of the weight off for at least one year. Curioni and Lourenço noted that approximately 50 percent of the weight lost was regained by all regardless of the method they used to lose weight. Part of the reason for this may be due to the fact that they also found those who lost more weight in the beginning of their weight loss efforts were not as effective at sustaining that loss. Although these researchers made note of the fact that most of the studies they included in their article were of poor quality, they concluded that the weight lost using diet and exercise translates into weight loss that would occur in everyday life outside of the context of a research study. By contrast, another group headed by Douketis concluded that while weight loss occurs the problems inherent in how the studies are designed prevent the findings from being applicable to a real-world setting.

Douketis and colleagues examined a group of studies that researched long-term weight loss as a result of behavioral changes, medication, and weight loss surgery. They reported that making behavioral changes such as dietary and lifestyle changes results in weight loss less than 11 pounds that is maintained for 2–4 years. Taking weight-loss medications (which can typically only be taken for a brief period of time) can result in weight loss between 11 pounds and 22 pounds that is maintained for 1–2 years, and weight-loss surgery can result in substantial weight loss (i.e., 55–165 pounds) that is maintained for 2–4 years. These researchers concluded that while these studies clearly show weight loss is maintained for a year or more depending on the weight loss method they added that these findings do not have clinical utility which means that the findings should not be used by health-care professionals or laypeople as recommendations for what they should do for weight loss. Douketis and colleagues noted that the vast majority of studies did not collect data after three years which they contrasted to studies examining chronic illnesses such as diabetes and hypertension which usually follow people from 4 to 8 years. Additionally, in studies where follow up was at 2 years the participant dropout rate ranged from 30 percent to 57 percent and in clinical trials (i.e., studies designed to determine if a particular treatment can be used in practice) the dropout rate should be less than 20 percent.

A study published in 2010 collected weight-related data on over 14,000 adults in the United States. The research group led by Jennifer Krashnewski of the Penn State College of Medicine used the long-term weight loss maintenance definition suggested by Wing and Hill of the National Weight Control Registry. Based on their findings they reported that over 36 percent of adults in their study maintained a 5 percent weight loss, over 17 percent maintained a 10 percent weight loss, 8.5 percent maintained a 15 percent weight loss, and just under 4.5 percent maintained a 20 percent weight loss. They noted that the proportion of participants that lost 10 percent is better than what is typically found in clinical trials which led them to conclude that adults seeking to achieve long-term weight loss maintenance might be more successful at it than other studies have previously indicated. They also noted that even though a significant proportion of adults were not able to achieve and maintain weight loss of any kind, the adults who did achieve and maintain weight loss should be studied more carefully to determine what they are doing that sets them apart from adults who are not able to lose weight and maintain that loss. They also noted that if whatever is learned from this group could be applied to those struggling to lose weight there would be great benefit to public health. Finally, Krashnewski and colleagues recognized the flaws of the study which included the idea that they do not know if weight cycling may have occurred in between the start of the study and follow up, or if weight regain was in process (participants may have gained weight but still maintained a certain percentage of weight loss), they also did not know how participants went about losing their weight which can mean that some weight loss may have been the result of illness, and all data was self-reported which can be unreliable.

A recent meta-analysis conducted by a group of researchers headed by Dombrowski was published in 2014 and summarized the findings from 45 highly controlled experiments that examined long-term weight loss as a result of non-surgical efforts (i.e., behavior changes and medications). They concluded this group of studies demonstrated that weight loss can occur via lifestyle changes and/or prescription medication and that weight regain is slowed for up to 12 months. At the two-year mark, however, the strength of this finding begins to weaken, and beyond 24 months there is limited evidence that weight regain will be minimized. While these findings are somewhat promising in terms of whether or not weight loss is possible, Dombrowski and colleagues noted that just under half of the studies they looked at did not report results from participants who dropped out of the study which meant they only had data on those who started and finished. They noted that pharmacological intervention may be effective for weight loss for up to three years; however, along with weight loss was an increase in unpleasant side effects (e.g., gastrointestinal issues) that may make this intervention less attractive to those outside of the context of a research study.

Numerous studies have examined whether or not long-term weight loss is possible. All of the studies examined here used the definition posited by Wing and Hill that someone who loses at least 10 percent of their overall body weight and keeps it off for at least one year they will have achieved long-term weight loss. Despite some researchers noting that caution should be taken in how the data are interpreted or ultimately used, they all concluded that long-term weight loss is possible and worth pursuing.

Long-Term Weight Loss Is Not Possible

Those who have criticized the statement that long-term weight loss is possible point to the idea that keeping weight off for one year does not constitute a time frame that is long term. They argue that weight loss maintained over five years is a more robust indicator of long-term weight loss. Moreover, some of these researchers question whether or not pursing weight loss in the first place is a good idea.

In a 2006 study on dieting behaviors in adolescents, Dianne Neumark-Sztainer and colleagues concluded that engaging in dieting behaviors can have the opposite result than what is intended: weight gain. They noted that several studies conducted over the course of several years had previously shown that weight gain followed dieting, but it was unclear what might explain this seemingly paradoxical trend. Dianne Neumark-Sztainer's group studied over 2500 male and female adolescents over the course of five years. They measured dieting behavior, binge eating, whether or not study participants ate breakfast, fruits, and vegetables, and whether or not they engaged in physical activity. They also measured BMI to determine if this changed from the initial measurement to the measurement taken five years later. All data collected were self-reported data, and while this type of data can be unreliable it is consistent with how other studies collect data related to dieting and weight loss.

Neumark-Sztainer and her colleagues concluded that what seemed to predict weight gain was not necessarily the dieting itself but other behaviors that are associated with or are the result of having gone on a diet. They explained that dieting or going on a diet is usually viewed as something that is done temporarily to solve a particular problem—in this case weight loss. Given that mind-set they suggested that instead of engaging in behaviors that might result in more effective weight management, they are more like to engage in yo-yo dieting which involves going on and off of diets. Overall, this study revealed that dieting was a strong predictor of engaging in binge eating behavior indicating that the more one dieted the more likely they were to eventually binge eat. Binge eating in turn was associated with and strongly predicted an increase in BMI over time. These researchers noted that the relationship between dieting and BMI is complex, and there are likely additional factors that may help to explain why dieting would be associated with a higher BMI several years later. Nonetheless, they concluded that the relationship between these two variables was strong indicating that more fully understanding the nature of the relationship between dieting and weight gain is an important line of scientific inquiry.

In 2006 Astrid Lang and Erika Sivarajan Froelicher examined the existing literature published in the medical field on long-term weight loss and maintenance. They found that when weight loss efforts were effective they included a combination of changes to eating and physical activity, and involved behavioral modification efforts (i.e., learning what reinforces certain behaviors in order to make effective behavior changes). They further concluded, however, that while weight loss in the short term seems to be routinely demonstrated, long-term maintenance of the initial weight lost was not something that can be counted on. Lang and Froelicher concluded by saying that obesity (and by contrast weight loss) is not an issue of willpower or a matter of self-control, rather it is something that is more complicated than that and involves behavioral and physiological factors. This view is consistent with the growing body of literature indicating that obesity has numerous causes including genetics and is not entirely within the control of the individual.

Another group of researchers lead by Traci Mann examined the studies that had been conducted in the area of weight loss to determine if weight loss should be recommended as a treatment for obesity. They applied the

GRADE (Grading of Recommendations, Assessment, Development and Evaluation) system of evaluating research which, according to the group's website, was developed for the purpose of helping health-care providers and policy makers determine whether or not a particular treatment method is effective and beneficial. As such, they recommend that research be evaluated in terms of the quality of the evidence, which involves how well the study was designed and carried out, when there are multiple outcomes a determination is made regarding which outcomes are most critical, the quality of the evidence among these important outcomes, and finally an evaluation of whether or not any benefits outweigh potential harm. The GRADE workgroup notes that conclusions based on existing evidence have a real and direct impact on whether or not a particular treatment is implemented since historically there is inconsistency worldwide with respect to rating the quality of evidence and the robustness of recommendations made based on that evidence. They further point out that when the quality of the evidence is not considered when making health-care recommendations some treatments may be erroneously recommended because the recommendation itself is based on poorly conducted research.

As an example they point to the long-standing recommendation that post-menopausal women be treated with hormone replacement therapy as it was shown in the research to reduce patient's risk of cardiovascular problems. The GRADE group pointed out that since then more rigorous research has shown that this treatment not only does not reduce the risk of cardiovascular events it may also place patients at greater risk for such events. Thus, this workgroup noted that if a rating system like the one they propose had been used to evaluate the previous research and subsequent recommendations in this area, the conclusion would likely have been that the evidence was not of high enough quality to make any recommendations on hormone-replacement therapy. Higher quality research conducted later would have demonstrated that there is the strong possibility of harm to patients should hormone replacement therapy be recommended. Examples such as this are offered as illustrations of why quality research is important when making treatment recommendations that will be implemented by health-care providers who dutifully read the research and follow the recommendations of their professional boards and organizations. As such, Traci Mann and her colleagues questioned whether or not the prevailing treatment recommendation for obesity which is weight loss or dieting (defined as the "severe restriction of calorie intake") was based on research that met the standards of the GRADE system. This group also focused their efforts on studies conducted on long-term weight loss since they pointed out that short-term weight loss is not truly a treatment for obesity.

Their initial conclusion was that dieting does, in fact, lead to short-term weight loss but that whatever is lost is not sustained long term. One of the studies they reviewed concluded that the issue is not whether or not weight regain occurs but how quickly it occurs. Traci Mann and her colleagues noted that the longer study participants were followed the more weight was regained indicating that a longer follow up is likely to reveal even more weight regained. In considering well-designed studies that used several groups, including a control group (a group that is not receiving the treatment, which in this case is a diet), Mann and her colleagues concluded that after two years the average sustained weight loss was just over 4.5 pounds, but when comparing the dieting group to the non-dieting group after three years there was no difference in weight and in fact overall there was a 3.5 pound weight gain.

In their evaluation of studies designed to make cause-and-effect conclusions about dieting (i.e., the studies that involve randomly assigning participants to one of two or more groups such as a diet group and a non-diet group), Traci Mann and her colleagues concluded that although the studies were well designed they did not reveal a substantial long-term weight loss leaving participants in the same weight category (i.e., obese) as when they started. They also noted that among the studies that examined health benefits of any weight loss it was not clear that dieting was the cause of these benefits. Confounding variables (i.e., factors that were not studied but that may explain the results) such as lower sodium intake and less alcohol consumed were not sufficiently examined and therefore a conclusion about what caused the benefits found in these studies could not be made.

Other studies that did not use comparison groups had low follow-up rates (an average of one-third of the participants did not complete the follow-up information) from the start of the study to up to five years later which can lead to data that shows dieting was more effective than it actually was. Many of these studies used self-reported weights which have routinely been shown in other research to be unreliable with participants consistently underestimating their weight by nearly five pounds and up to just over eight pounds. Most of the studies examined by Mann's research group did not account for the impact exercise may have had on the results. Research consistently shows those who included exercise in their efforts are more successful at sustaining weight loss. Traci Mann and her colleagues note, however, that since the intent was to evaluate the effectiveness of dieting then other factors such as exercise should have been methodologically controlled so that the effect of dieting alone could have been determined. Finally, it was reported that in a subset of these studies a meaningful percentage of participants (from 20 percent to 65 percent) had engaged in at least one and in some cases up to three other diets since the start of the study resulting in additional weight loss. While participating in other forms of diets means that the participants are engaged in dieting (which is the purpose of the study), this affects the quality of the study since the intent is to study the effectiveness of the original diet, not serial dieting which when not accounted for can make the original diet look more effective than it actually is.

The final group of studies this group examined is referred to as prospective studies. These studies involved recruiting people who chose to diet and people who chose not to diet, which means that participants were not assigned to a dieting condition or a non-dieting condition. Data were collected at the start of the study and again at designated follow-up times. The group noted that very few studies conducted in this way took into account confounding variables such as exercise. Of the studies Mann's group examined, one showed that dieting led to weight loss over time, two studies did not find a connection between dieting and weight loss, and seven studies demonstrated that dieting led to weight gain.

When examining the findings of the research looking at whether or not dieting leads to weight loss, the final consideration to make using the GRADE system is to compare the benefits identified with the treatment to potential harm associated with the treatment. Traci Mann and her colleagues concluded that the benefits identified associated with dieting are small and those that were found may not in fact be the result of dieting but may be the result of other factors such as low sodium intake, engaging in exercise, or effects of medication prescribed to treat hypertension. Additionally, most of studies demonstrated that the majority of dieters will regain most if not all of the weight they lost and some will exceed the weight they were at the start of the study. This, in combination with the finding in some studies that a substantial percentage of participant engaged in more than one form of diet, led this group to point to the danger of weight cycling (aka yo-yo dieting), which is common among dieters and has been associated with its own group of problems such as a higher mortality rate, death from cardiovascular disease, greater risk of diabetes, stroke and high blood pressure, and a compromised immune system. Overall, Traci Mann and her colleagues concluded that the benefits of dieting do not outweigh the potential for harm and therefore suggest that dieting should not be recommended as a treatment for obesity.

One of the things contributing to the debate regarding weight loss (i.e., whether or not can it occur long term and whether or not it results in health benefits) involves whether or not the research conducted was done in a methodologically sound manner. That is, was the research conducted in such a way that it is clear what may have led to the outcomes of the study? In this case, is it clear that dieting is what led to weight loss (as opposed to something else like exercise)? Is it clear that dieting and subsequent weight loss is the reason for any health benefits (as opposed to something like exercise, or consuming less sodium)? While there is evidence to suggest that weight loss may be possible for many people in the short term and for some people in the long term, others have identified significant issues with the design and conclusions of these studies calling into question the conclusion that long-term weight loss is truly possible.

BODY SIZE AND LIFE EXPECTANCY

As discussed in the earlier section Diseases Linked to Obesity, there have been many diseases connected to obesity that raised concerns about life expectancy and longevity. Certainly if someone is at greater risk for cancer, diabetes, hypertension, and other cardiovascular issues, they are at greater risk of having a shorter life-span than if they were not at risk for developing those diseases. As noted in the Diseases Linked to Obesity section, there are questions regarding whether or not it is obesity that places someone at greater risk for these medical issues or if factors other than obesity (e.g., metabolic syndrome) may be the cause. Given the presumed link between obesity and an earlier death because obesity is linked to many serious diseases, and given the question about whether or not obesity is truly the risk factor of concern, it is not surprising that research has been conducted to examine whether or not body size affects life expectancy.

In 2009, a study conducted by the Prospective Studies Collaboration compared BMI to cause-specific mortality (i.e., what specifically caused someone's death). This group was interested in determining whether or not BMI was an important factor in predicting and explaining mortality. They examined 57 studies that had previously collected data on mortality, mortality risk factors, and BMI. They intended to determine what these studies collectively showed with respect to the relationship between BMI and mortality. In total, the 57 studies had data from nearly 900,000 adults primarily in North America and Western Europe. Based on the findings of these studies, this research collaboration concluded that the lowest mortality rate was found among those with a BMI between 22.5 and 25, which spans from the middle of the normal weight category to the lowest point on the overweight category according to WHO's BMI classification system. They also noted that for every increase of 5 BMI points there was a 30 percent higher risk of all-cause mortality indicating that the higher one's BMI above the normal range the more likely one is to die. They also found, however, that a BMI below the normal range, which would be classified by the WHO as underweight, produced an inverse relationship with mortality meaning that the lower the BMI in this range the higher the mortality risk. This group noted that since BMI is not a perfect measure of where fat is stored in the body it is likely that the mortality rate is even higher among those who are overweight or obese than their findings demonstrate. Interestingly, a study conducted in Demark over the course of nearly four decades offered results that may, in part, contradict the findings of this 2009 study.

A study conducted in Denmark and published in 2016 in the *Journal of the American Medical Association* examined the BMI of those who died between 1976 and 1978, 1991 and 1994, and 2003and 2013. These researchers were interested in determining what BMI had the lowest mortality rate and whether or not that has changed over nearly four decades. The data was collected via the Copenhagen City Heart Study during the 1970s and 1990s data collection periods, and via the Copenhagen General Population Study during the 2000s to 2010s period. Data were available on 13,704 individuals during the 1970s period, 9,482 during the 1990s, and 97,362 during the 2000s to 2010s period. At the final follow up in 2014 78 percent, 53 percent, and 6 percent of those who participated the 1970s, 1990s, and 2000s to 2010s studies, respectively, had died.

When examining who had the lowest mortality rate in terms of BMI, the researchers found that BMI and its accompanying classification in terms of obesity have risen over the years. In the 1970s, those with a BMI of 23.7 had the lowest all-cause mortality (i.e., death by any cause). This BMI is categorized as being in the normal range according to WHO's weight classification system. In the 1990s, the BMI with the lowest mortality had risen slightly to 24.6, which is still within the normal range of the WHO classification system. Finally, during 2000s to 2010s, the BMI with the lowest all-cause mortality was 27.0, which is categorized as overweight or pre-obese. The highest mortality rates in this population were found among those with the lowest and highest BMIs.

The researchers noted that the explanation for why the trend of a higher BMI associated with the lowest all-cause mortality risk has occurred is not known. They suggested that it is possible the improvements in treatment of the risk factors for cardiovascular disease have improved such that there is a reduced mortality for all classes of BMI but that the greatest impact may have been on those with a higher BMI. They also noted that public health campaigns that have targeted smoking habits and physical activity may also account for the findings. Regardless of the reason for the findings, it is likely surprising to many that the most recent data collected in this study indicates that being overweight may mean that your mortality risk is lower when compared to those who are underweight, obese, or normal weight.

A concern raised in some of these studies was examined explicitly by James Greenberg in a study published in 2006. He noted that a condition called *reverse causality* may increase the mortality risk found among low BMIs (i.e., underweight), which if not corrected can result in a lower mortality rate among those with higher BMIs. Reverse causality refers to a cause-and-effect finding that is the opposite of what would be expected. In this case, the expected finding would be that the higher one's BMI the higher the risk for death and the lower one's BMI the lower the risk for death. The reverse causality finding in this case is reflected in studies that have regularly found that there is a high rate of mortality among people with low BMI. Researchers such as Greenberg, who express concern about such a finding, indicated that it may not be BMI that is causal factor of death in the underweight classification, rather the causal factor is a disease process which can cause both death and weight loss. Therefore, in his analysis he only included participants who did not have a history of serious illness which could result in death and weight loss including heart disease, stroke, cancer, or emphysema. He also excluded people who stated that they had limitations in their activities of daily living. As a result of his analysis, which eliminated the reverse causality bias, Greenberg found that excess deaths (i.e., deaths that have a specific cause due to disease or some other conditions that would cause one's death) associated with obesity increased by 313 percent.

Greenberg's decision to examine reverse causality was made in part due to a study published in 2005 by a research team led by Katherine Flegal. Flegal and her colleagues found a lower number of deaths than expected that were attributable to obesity. They surmised that their low estimates may have been due in part to the fact that they did not examine whether or not there were any other factors (such as disease) that might cause both death and a lower BMI. As noted above, Greenberg concluded that low estimates such as those found by Flegal's group are probably due to exactly that. Eight years later in 2013, Flegal headed another research group that reviewed the existing research in the area of all-cause mortality and BMI classification. They conducted a meta-analysis to determine the degree to which certain BMI categories may be at risk for higher rates of mortality. They confirmed higher BMIs, specifically BMIs of 35 or higher, were at risk for higher all-cause mortality when compared to those who are normal weight. However, her group also found that a BMI of 30–34.00

(Grade I Obesity) was not associated with higher mortality and confirmed the findings of others that showed the lowest all-cause mortality rate was found among those in the overweight category. Moreover, Flegal and her colleagues concluded that their results did not support the idea that a pre-existing illness would bias their findings. The self-report nature of the data was, however, a limitation, which is found in most studies examining these issues.

Mark Hamer and Emmanuel Stamatakis examined whether or not there was a difference between metabolically healthy and metabolically unhealthy obese individuals in terms of the risk for cardiovascular disease—which is a leading cause of death worldwide. These researchers included over 22,000 men and women in their study who at the time the study began did not have a history of cardiovascular disease. They collected a number of measurements including BMI to determine whether or not study participants were obese, data to determine the metabolic health of the participants (e.g., diabetes diagnosis, degree of inflammation), and when a study participant died they collected the cause of death information. Among the 22,000+ study participants, just under 24 percent were classified as obese and among this group nearly 25 percent of these participants were classified as metabolically healthy. By contrast, 33 percent or one-third of the nonobese participants were classified as metabolically unhealthy. Over the course of the multi-year study 2472 participants died with 604 who died as a result of cardiovascular disease and 1868 were all-cause deaths. In order to determine who was at greater risk of death, Hamer and Stamatakis compared the obese to the nonobese and the metabolically healthy to the non-metabolically healthy. They found that the metabolically healthy obese were at no greater risk of cardiovascular disease when compared to the metabolically healthy nonobese; however, when either the obese or nonobese participants had two or more indicators of being metabolically unhealthy, both groups were at greater risk of cardiovascular disease. Their final conclusion was that the metabolically healthy obese were not at greater risk of cardiovascular disease or all-cause mortality over a seven-year period. They further stated that in aggregate, their results indicated it is not adiposity (being fat) that predicts cardiovascular disease or other deaths; rather it is one's overall metabolic health.

Overall, the research discussed in this chapter sheds light on the fact that conclusions drawn based on obesity, health, and mortality ought to be done with care. There is a growing body of research contradicting the long-standing position that having a larger body automatically means that person is unhealthy or that they will die sooner than their smaller bodied counterparts. This research indicates that it may not be weight itself that is the factor of interest when it comes to why some people get certain diseases and others do not but one's overall metabolic health. Additionally, it may be that being overweight or even mildly obese is a protective factor when it comes to early death.

CHAPTER 8

Is Personal Choice a Relevant Argument for Body Size?

When obesity is written about or reported about on the news, it is often accompanied by such phrases as "the obesity epidemic" or the "obesity crisis," and at times obesity is referred to as a "global health crisis." As such, obesity and even overweight are seen as conditions or diseases to be reduced or eliminated altogether. Many have argued that due to numerous diseases linked to obesity it is not only a burden to the individual and his or her loved ones, but it is a burden to the populace at large. Those who take this stance have pointed to the findings that indicate obesity as a financially costly disease and part of what has driven the rise in the cost of health care including treatment, health-care insurance, and life insurance. Critics of this position have pointed to the research noted in previous sections of this book (e.g., it is not obesity but other conditions that are linked to the medical diseases associated with obesity) as evidence that obesity is not a problem and therefore not a burden to society at large. Critics have also indicated that given the growing body of research supporting the idea that obesity is not likely the cause of various medical diseases we should focus more on the diseases themselves and what causes them (since they are also found in non-obese individuals) rather than on body size which is the result of the complex interaction of genetics, environment, and personal choices. This section will examine the degree to which obesity may or may not affect the public at large, and even if it does, what role personal choice plays in this issue.

What Are the Costs of Obesity for Everyone?

The correlation between obesity and numerous health-related issues is one area of concern that has seemingly prompted health-care providers, policy makers, and educators to develop programs designed to eliminate obesity. An additional area of concern often cited for the need for these programs is the overall financial cost of obesity, which is assumed to be passed on to the general public.

Obesity is considered to be a worldwide epidemic by the World Health Organization. The Centers for Disease Control and Prevention (CDC) concurs with respect to the prevalence of obesity in the United States. As of 2015, no state in the United States had an obesity prevalence rate among adults of less than 20 percent, and four states had a prevalence rate of 35 percent or more. For children ages 2–19 years old, the prevalence rate across the United States was 17 percent with rates as high as nearly 22 percent among Hispanic youth and as low as 8.6 percent among non-Hispanic Asian youth.

According to the group The State of Obesity, estimates for health-care costs and treatment of chronic diseases for those who are obese are thought to be around $150 billion to over $200 billion. Overall, adults who are obese are believed to pay around 42 percent more for overall health care than adults with a healthy BMI. For those with a BMI of 40 or higher, it is estimated that the cost of health care is over 80 percent higher in comparison to adults with a healthy BMI. The State of Obesity also noted that with the implementation of evidence-based community prevention efforts nearly $7 billion could be saved by Medicare and Medicaid combined.

According to the Campaign to End Obesity, a governmental group called the Congressional Budget Office reported in 2010 that not only had there been a measurable increase in health-care costs from 1987 to 2007 but 20 percent of that increase in cost was caused by obesity. This finding was based on calculations looking at changes in rates of obesity and health-care costs over that 20-year period. They noted that a greater number of people became obese during that time period than in previous time periods. They surmised that if the rate of obesity had remained as in earlier years then health-care costs would have been 20 percent lower than they were by 2007. This same report showed that there was 80 percent increase in overall health-care expenditures from 1987 to 2007. Some of that increase in spending was explained by more people having insurance coverage, by an increase in the older adult population, new more expensive medical technology, and the fact that medical treatment simply costs more even after adjusting for inflation. All weight categories demonstrated an overall increase in health-care spending but that expenditures were the highest among those who were classified as obese. They reported that there was a 65 percent increase in health-care spending among normal weight individuals and a 111 percent increase among obese individuals.

A study conducted in 2013 and published in the *Clinical Obesity* journal examined what contributed to the cost of obesity by looking at health-care-related databases that included medical claims filed with insurance companies. Consistent with other reports, the authors of this study found that obesity was associated with a high degree of expenditure. They noted that since obesity has been routinely identified as associated with conditions such as diabetes and hypertension then it would follow that reducing the prevalence of obesity would also reduce health-care costs for the disease linked to obesity. They also indicated that an important explanation for the higher costs was the higher rate of inpatient admissions compared to their lower weight counterparts. Inpatient treatment suggests that whatever the medical concerns are they are significant enough that they cannot be treated in an outpatient health-care setting (e.g., the doctor's office) and therefore required 24-hour monitoring, which is expensive.

Anne Dee and her colleagues examined not only the direct costs associated with obesity (e.g., paying for health-care procedures) but also indirect costs (e.g., loss of productivity at work). In line with what others have reported, they found that as BMI increases so do costs of health-care as well as costs due to loss of work-related productivity. They further concluded that the indirect costs were higher than those associated with direct health-care expenditures. They looked at numerous studies and determined that there were such significant differences in how these studies were conducted that conclusions drawn from and policies based on these findings should be done with caution. These authors also concluded that if these findings are used to develop treatment recommendations or to establish health-care policy they should be subsequently evaluated in terms of their cost-effectiveness. Thus, if health-care policies, community-based programs, or health-care interventions are developed based on the finding that larger body sizes, particularly obese bodies, have greater costs associated with them then it needs to be determined if these efforts have the kind of impact (e.g., lower costs, higher productivity) that makes such efforts worthwhile.

Critics of the position that obesity costs taxpayers more money either through the increased cost in specific procedures or the increased cost of health-care premiums point to several factors that suggest these presumed costs could be eliminated not through eliminating obesity but through addressing the underlying causes of various diseases and by changing how the obese are treated by people in general and by health-care providers in particular.

Although obesity has been linked to a variety of diseases (e.g., cardiovascular disease, diabetes), recent research has indicated that these diseases may not develop as a result of increased weight per se, but the manner in which weight is stored. That is, not all fatty tissue is stored the same way which has a direct impact on overall health. Moreover, there are metabolic indicators that predict some of these diseases and these metabolic issues can be found among people of all weights including upward of 30 percent of those at a normal weight. Additionally, these metabolic issues are also found to predict weight gain. Thus, critics point to the idea that blaming obesity or obese people for the reported rise in health-care costs is inaccurate. That it is not obesity itself that gives rise to these diseases, but other factors that predict both many of the diseases and weight itself. Therefore, singling out overweight and obesity is believed to be inappropriate and inaccurate.

Regardless, some people have argued that those who are obese should pay more in health-care premiums since they cost more to treat—that this cost should not be shared, rather it should be borne by those who are the cause of such increases. Critics of this position indicate that if in fact obesity is driving up health-care costs for everyone then we also need to single out other demographics or behaviors that may result in costly injury or disease. For example, they suggest that if we are prepared to demand that those who are obese take on more of the burden of the cost of health-care, then we ought to also single out people who engage in risky behaviors such as athletes (who are prone to regular injury), motorcycle riders (especially those who do not wear helmets), or for that matter those who ride in or drive a car regularly since that form of travel is known to be much more dangerous than air travel.

Certainly, the overall increase in the cost of health-care is felt by nearly all who carry health-care insurance or who pay for health-care services directly. Thus, it is certainly normal to want to not pay for any more than one has to. Moreover, if there is an identifiable group that has been connected to increased costs that are felt by millions of people then it too is normal to demand that they are the one who pay for such an increase. If obesity truly is a causal factor in the rise in health-care costs, what if there are other factors contributing to one's obesity or diseases related to obesity that cause the presumed hike in health-care costs? What if how those who are obese are treated is the reason for increased costs?

As has been previously discussed, anti-fat bias, the stigma of obesity, and shame-based prevention efforts (see Chapter 4) have been strongly linked to mental health concerns including things like low self-esteem, depression, and anxiety. These are all costly issues not only in terms of the mental toll it takes on those dealing with them, but also physically given the link between mental well-being and overall physical health, and they are costly financially to treat. Critics of the idea that obese individuals should bear a greater financial burden for rising health-care costs note that prevention efforts ought not to be focused on reducing obesity but on reducing bullying and other forms of oppression both of which are linked to serious mental and physical health problems. They note that by intervening on that level it is likely that those who are obese will feel less stigmatized, less demoralized, and display fewer cases of mental and physical health problems.

Finally, critics of efforts to target obese individuals point to the research indicating that health-care providers themselves bear some of the same attitudes that the general public has. Health-care providers have been found to have an anti-fat bias that is not as prevalent as that among the general population but that is measureable and likely to negatively impact the treatment obese individuals receive. In comparison to their more normal weight peers, obese individuals often get less time with their health-care providers, are more likely to be told to lose weight rather than be told about interventions specifically designed to address their medical concern, and are less likely to receive education around regular prevention efforts. Additionally, when an obese individual is not physically comfortable (e.g., waiting room chairs that do not accommodate their size) or mentally comfortable (e.g., they are told to lose weight for nearly every concern that brings them to the doctor's office), they are less likely to visit their health-care professional, which means they are not getting the treatment they need to address any mental health or medical concerns that may be caught and treated early on resulting in fewer costs. They are also less likely to have routine check-ups or prevention screens which can also result in disease processes not identified or treated, which will then be likely to ultimately cost more in the long run.

Critics question the veracity that obese individuals are the cause of rising health-care costs. It is clear that health-care costs have in fact risen over the years, but the causes of those increases may have more to do with factors that do not include body size or any other such personal factor. Even if obesity is a factor in the rising health-care costs then critics suggest that dealing with stigmatization of larger body sizes would result in fewer health-related problems and better overall health care, which may have an impact on overall health-care costs. Regardless of whether or not there is a connection between obesity and rising health-care costs, some question whether or not an obese person is responsible to the larger society such that he or she is obligated to attain a smaller body no matter what.

PERSONAL RESPONSIBILITY OR SHARED RESPONSIBILITY?

There is little doubt that most adults in developed countries have autonomy and therefore choice with respect to what they eat and what exercise they engage in. Where there is debate, however, is in terms of whether or not we have a choice with regard to body size. Two adults eating the same types and quantities of food, and engaging in the same type, quantity, and intensity of exercise will not weigh the same even if they are of the same sex, same age, and same height. As has been discussed in previous sections, there are other factors besides eating and exercise behaviors that contribute to body shape and size. Nonetheless, given the research linking obesity to numerous health issues and statistics connecting obesity to increased monetary costs, there are some who advocate for the position that those who are overweight have an obligation if not a duty to become a smaller size. Accompanying that stance is the belief that a smaller body size will result in better health and lower costs. Whether or not that is true still begs the question of whether or not we are allowed to decide for ourselves how we live our lives, no matter what size our body is? There are those who suggest that freedom of choice should be maintained but add that those making bad choices should be held responsible for those choices. Others have indicated that those making bad (i.e., unhealthy) food choices are weak willed and do not have the discipline necessary to resist tempting and well-advertised food.

In his article examining the role responsibility plays in obesity, Benjamin Brooks argues for a shared or social responsibility for obesity rather placing it on the individual. He suggests that the government plays a role in regulating food availability and food choice which ultimately influences personal choices. By saying that personal responsibility should be applied to obesity and by extension to obese individuals, this redirects the focus off any role the government or the public at large may play. He suggests that obesity prevention should be considered in the context of shared responsibility and that all involved should examine in what way they contribute to promoting or combating obesity.

Further muddying the waters, according to Wendy Mariner a professor of Health Law at Boston University, is health insurance and how it contributes to defining who is responsible for health. She notes that focusing on the cost of medical services has led to cost-sharing in insurance which further gives rise to the idea that health and well-being is the responsibility of the individual rather than the responsibility of the society in which that individual lives. That is, if someone has to have an expensive medical procedure, their insurance will cover the cost of that, but because they had an expensive medical procedure there may be a subsequent rise in what everyone pays in insurance premiums. So, someone who does not need expensive medical care will effectively share the cost of that person's medical care by paying the same insurance premium. This reality, that some people need more medical care than others, has led many to declare that it is not fair, and that people who need more medical care should be responsible for that not only through their lifestyle choices but also by paying more for insurance. And, by contrast, those who need less medical care should pay less. Therefore, anyone who is obese should be required to pay more or take action to get their weight under control.

It is not surprising that many people take the position that body weight is well within someone's control. We hear this from our medical providers who tell us to lose weight regardless of the reason for our visit, and we hear it repeatedly in the media we consume. A study published in the *Medical Journal of Australia* examined how news and stories presented via television depict overweight and obesity. The authors found that an overwhelming majority (72%) of the media-related items portrayed obesity as a result of poor nutrition and 66 percent of the items depicted obesity as being under the control of the individual. The authors concluded that television stories and news items may help perpetuate the notion that obesity is the fault of the individual. Moreover, they noted that since this is a problem to be solved by individuals they found that any solutions presented for the obesity problem revolved around individual willpower to control one's appetite or to engage in more physical activity. Therefore, the message is clear: if you are obese it is your fault, and only you can fix it.

Many of those who are unsympathetic to the experiences of people who are overweight or obese are often of the mind that whatever ills they experience, physical or psychological, they have brought it on themselves. They believe since the size and shape of one's body is entirely within one's control, then any ill effects of having a larger body is that person's fault. If an obese child is being bullied for his or her size, then the solution is to lose weight. If someone has diabetes then, again, the solution is to lose weight. When the answer to any problem connected to weight is to lose weight, the underlying assumption is that gaining or losing weight is entirely within any person's control, and whatever size they are, it is their responsibility or fault. This notion is the focus of an article written by Bruce Waller entitled "Responsibility and Health." In his article, Mr. Waller notes that taking responsibility for one's health and further being responsible for one's health status are often conflated when they are actually two distinct ideas. He refers to the former as *take-charge respon-sibility* and the later as *just-deserts responsibility.*

Making autonomous decisions for one's life and health has been found to be beneficial to both mind and body. When we feel like we have the freedom to choose and make decisions that are best for us, we are healthier both physically and mentally. By contrast, if our ability to make autono-mous decisions is limited or taken away completely, both our physical and mental health suffer. Thus, in his article on responsibility and health, Mr. Waller notes that autonomy, or personal responsibility in health care, is something that should be encouraged. He noted that we should be allowed to make decisions for ourselves based on our abilities and information we have available to us. This will mean, of course, that some of us will make decisions that are objectively healthier than others, which leads to the con-cern about whether or not we should also be responsible for the outcomes of our decisions.

Mr. Waller states that the conflation of take-charge responsibility (we should be in charge of our health-care) and just-deserts responsibility (deserving praise or blame for our actions depending on the outcome) can lead to things like learned helplessness, loss of self-efficacy, and overall drop in motivation to make healthy decisions for one's self. Mr. Waller discusses this issue in terms of whether or not it is fair to apply health-related benefits such as who gets access to organ donations, or other scarce medical resources on the basis of decisions that someone makes that may or may not have a positive outcome. For example, should someone who has been a chronic drinker be denied a liver because of the decisions he has made? Many people, including health-care providers, would say yes because this person chose to drink, which resulted in a damaged liver, therefore, he is less deserving than the person with liver disease who was not a chronic drinker. Mr. Waller challenges this notion by encouraging readers to move beyond immediately observable behaviors and consider what may or may not have contributed to someone's ability to make health decisions.

For example, he noted that a student who works really hard only to get average grades does not get nearly the accolades as the student who is nat-urally gifted, rarely puts in any effort yet gets excellent grades. Similarly, he points to the example of a man who while growing up was not encour-aged to take careful consideration of decisions he was making. Rather, those around him impatiently expected him to make decisions or take action quickly without carefully contemplating outcomes. Thus, as a man with take-charge responsibility for his health care, he is much more likely to make impulsive decisions without taking the time to carefully consider how his decisions may or may not affect his overall health. Mr. Waller then asks whether or not it is fair to require this man to wait to receive the needed health-care in deference to those who made better and healthier decisions because they were taught early in their lives how to do so. He suggests that the first man did the best he could and was not given the tools needed in order to make healthier decisions. He further suggests that taking a morally based stance like just-deserts responsibility (he deserves the negative health consequences he gets and has to wait for health-care because of the choices he made) unfairly penalizes someone who could not have behaved any differently, and equally unfairly rewards those who may have been raised in an environment that encouraged healthy behaviors or who had the genetics that resisted chronic disease regardless of lifestyle.

Although Mr. Waller's article examines health-care in general and uses an example such as drinking to illustrate his ideas, it is not a stretch to transpose these examples with obesity. Given the multitude of factors, including genetics, that have an impact on body size, is it reasonable to differentially reward people based on outcome (i.e., just-deserts) rather than on healthy behaviors regardless of outcome? Surely if one takes the position that weight and health are inextricably linked and weight is under one's control then the outcome matters. A take-responsibility approach would simply say that each of us is responsible for our own health-care decisions, but that we cannot possibly be responsible for whether or not we achieve specific results—weight loss, improved health, and so on. There are simply too many variables that may facilitate or impede our ability to be healthy or lose weight despite our best efforts.

SHOULD ANYTHING BE DONE TO ENSURE PEOPLE DO NOT BECOME OBESE?

Those who work tirelessly to figure out what can be done to reduce the rate of obesity rely on the position that obesity is the direct result of human behavior. That is, if behaviors change then body size will change. However, many who devote attention to this area acknowledge that genetics are at play with respect to body size as are things like the manufacturing and processing of foods in developed countries, and an increasingly sedentary lifestyle supported in part by technological advances (i.e., gadgets and machinery that make many tasks easier); however, proposed efforts designed to address obesity are often focused on making individuals behave differently.

In 2013, Daniel Callahan published an article entitled *Obesity: Chasing an Elusive Epidemic*. In it he discusses the changes in rates of overweight and obesity as well as the efforts that have attempted to address weight loss. His position is that the weight loss efforts tried, to date, have largely been unsuccessful in that when weight-loss occurs it is only around 5–10 percent of one's body weight and in many cases the weight loss is not maintained. He therefore suggests that efforts to prevent people from becoming obese may need to come from the government and large business that target children and rely on social pressure.

Some efforts from governmental agencies have been attempted but, as Callahan noted, have been met with strong opposition from the public as well as powerful lobbying efforts. For example, when government officials in New York attempted to tax and limit the size of sugared drinks, they were met with strong opposition from food and agricultural lobbyists. The argument against such policies was reportedly framed in terms of allowing individuals the ability to choose what they wanted to consume, but Callahan and others have pointed out that such restrictions on food products would likely impact the bottom line of major food and agricultural businesses costing them billions in revenue. Businesses have seemingly had a bit more success in implementing policies related to body size by way of offering incentives and disincentives based on engaging or not engaging in healthy behavior. Some businesses have pledged to reduce sodium content in their food and others have pledged to reduce the cost of healthier foods. Critics of these efforts, however, note that such moves will only be made if the impact on the bottom line is either minimal or guaranteed to improve revenue.

Other companies have implemented efforts targeting their employees by rewarding (e.g., prizes, decrease in insurance premiums) them for successful healthy behaviors measured by weight loss, and by punishing (e.g., increase in insurance premiums) those who do engaged in those behaviors and lose weight. Callahan noted that it is possible that businesses may need to take a more coercive position by sending the message to their employees that they must engage in healthy behaviors or they will no longer be employed there but added that this begs the question of at what point are businesses helping and what point have they stepped over the line and are infringing on individuals' civil rights?

As for efforts focused on children, Callahan observed that there is a built-in mechanism for the kind of coercion discussed in the context of government and business: parents. He noted that the relationship between parent and child is such that parents have authority over their children and therefore can coerce or cajole them into engaging in healthy behaviors. But, he acknowledged, that parents need to buy into the idea that behaviors intended to prevent weight gain or result in weight loss are worthwhile since there is only so much that institutions like schools can do if the parents do not support these efforts at home. With respect to efforts beyond the family, Callahan noted that there have been some efforts to restrict how food is advertised to children both on school ground and via the media. He ultimately concludes that the most effective efforts may need to come from the government which can impose taxes and establish regulations targeting products believed to contribute to obesity.

The final way that Callahan believes obesity should be targeted is via social pressure. He makes the argument that since obesity causes disease, shortens one's lifespan (see Chapter 7 for a discussion of these issues), and is a factor in rising health-care costs, those who are obese need to recognize that they are part of the national health-care problem and global epidemic. If obese individuals cannot see this then, Callahan concludes, it is up to society at large to ensure that they do see this and make changes so they are no longer obese. According to him, an effective strategy would need to involve convincing obese individuals that healthy eating and exercise are good for them as well as those around them. This strategy would need to ensure that obesity is no longer socially acceptable, and the public would need to support government intervention to prevent and eliminate obesity even if those efforts are invasive or somewhat coercive. A part of these efforts, he says, should involve stigmatization which has a proven track record given campaigns against smoking.

Callahan clearly has taken the position that something needs to be done and soon. He believes that due to the seriousness of the epidemic, obesity needs to be eliminated and prevented at nearly any cost—including what he termed efforts that may be construed as coercive. Many people, researchers and lay people, are likely to agree with the idea that something needs to be done as soon as possible. And some may agree that if it takes coercion to make change happen then so be it. This, however, speaks to heart of personal choice and how far a society should go to change someone's behavior who has no interest in or is having difficulty with making such a change. Harald Schmidt examined Callahan's proposals and while he does not disagree with the ideas present outright, he does note that implementing programs designed to promote health and well-being is more complex than what Callahan and others may suggest.

Schmidt tested whether or not people would accept insurance penalties or incentives based on health-related behaviors. Overall, he did find that people seem to accept the idea of penalizing those who engage in behaviors that put their health at risk though they did not think the penalty should be too high. Based on these findings and his analysis of Callahan's proposed programs, Schmidt concluded that personal choice and responsibility is complicated. There is no one-size-fits-all approach that is likely to have the desired outcome of weight loss or the prevention of weight gain. He also stated that when larger, more systematic efforts are put in place, existing and proposed programs need to be evaluated in terms of the degree to which the programs are fair and refrain from blaming the victim, which in this case would be someone who is obese.

It is important to note, that both Callahan's and Schmidt's ideas with respect to obesity take the perspective that obesity is something that needs to be eliminated or prevented due to its connection with various diseases and rising health-care costs. As has been presented earlier (see Chapter 7), not everyone shares this perspective and some research directly contradicts this position. While they would likely agree with the idea of ensuring that programs are fair and don't focus on blame, and that promoting healthy behaviors is important, they would also argue that promotion of such behaviors should not have a specific demographic target. Moreover, they would point to research indicating that though obesity has been associated with many serious diseases, recent research has pointed to the notion that it is not body weight that is the causal factor but underlying metabolic issues that can be present in people regardless of body shape and size.

OBESITY AND THE LAW

As was discussed in the previous section, many people have the belief that something should be and needs to be done in order to prevent obesity from happening to begin with and to ensure those who are obese lose weight so they are no longer obese. In the current section, the issue of whether or not obesity is something that should be controlled via the legal system is discussed. Most of the arguments for legislating body size surround the issues of public health. Proponents of this approach point to the success previous legislation has had in reducing exposure to lead, rates of smoking, workplace safety, and overall vaccination rates. The suggestion now is that obesity needs to be added to the list of health issues that require legal intervention for the benefit of the general public.

Before getting into the specifics of law as it relates to obesity, it is useful to briefly examine the role the law plays in public health in general. A two-part article series entitled *Law as a Tool for Preventing Chronic Diseases: Expanding the Spectrum of Effective Public Health Strategies*, published by the CDC, examines this issue from the perspective of preventing chronic diseases. They note that there are two primary aims of the United States' national public health efforts which are to (1) improve quality of life as well as longevity and (2) to eliminate the disparities that exist with regard to rates of diseases among certain demographics and access to services. For chronic diseases, the authors of these articles indicate that the approach needs to be broad and include efforts focused on prevention, control of diseases and risk factors, and changes at the individual level, in the environment, in clinical services, and within organizations. As such, implementing these various approaches in the service of overall public health goals requires a massive systemic effort to determine what efforts need to be strengthened, replaced, eliminated, or changed. They argue that the law plays a pivotal role in these efforts.

Laws can be put in place at the national and/or state level levels to ensure that sufficient programs and policies are in place within health-care settings to ensure a level of care that will facilitate the goals of quality and length of life and ensuring that all citizens have equal access to services. Laws can be introduced that require behavior change by individuals (e.g., it is against the law to text and drive). Other laws may involve making changes to the environment such as putting fluoride in drinking water. Still other laws may impose requirements on organizations that result in behavior change such as a requirement to provide services designed to help people quit smoking. While these and other laws have had a positive impact on reducing rates of some chronic diseases, the authors of the CDC articles point out that laws alone cannot prevent or eliminate such diseases. They note that getting laws enacted is not usually an easy or quick process and that when they are put in place application of the laws and enforcement of them will vary. Thus, they concluded that laws should be considered one tool among many to address chronic health issues which may include obesity.

Michelle Mello and her colleagues examined the issues surrounding public health law and its role in obesity. They noted that previous public health efforts that have resulted in governmental and legal intervention (e.g., alcohol and smoking) have had a scientific basis for the existence of a public health crisis, and that there was accompanying social disapproval for the issues in question. They indicate that this is currently the situation with obesity which they say has resulted the public's desire for governmental involvement in and regulation of obesity. They also point to the American Medical Association's relatively recent classification of obesity as a disease in its own right as bolstering the evidence that something needs to be done beyond individuals taking personal responsibility for their body size. With respect to governmental involvement, Mello's group noted that in an opinion poll participants indicated they would most like the government to regulate how certain products are marketed to kids. They cited the arguments made when the tobacco industry was ordered to change their marketing campaigns. This included the idea that anything known to be or believed to be unhealthy should not be marketed toward children who do not have the capacity to fully process what they are exposed to and therefore cannot make healthy decisions. They are likely to be drawn to what looks or sounds good to them rather than whether or not it is good for them.

Because of concern for the health and well-being of children some programs have been highly criticized and some situations have resulted in formal lawsuits. For example, McDonald's was sued by obese children in New York for deceptive marketing practices and for not disclosing the risks associated with eating their food. Companies that manufacture and market soft drinks have been sued for similar reasons. Schools have been criticized for putting together lunch programs that are higher in saturated fats and sodium than is recommended by federal guidelines. Some states have proposed or initiated a junk food tax or fat tax with the idea that if junk foods are taxed people will be less likely to buy them, consume them, and ultimately become overweight or obese. There is no evidence, however, that this type of taxation will result in lower rates of obesity.

At the federal level, initiatives have been proposed that would regulate how unhealthy foods are marketed to children. This would include when they are marketed during children's television programming. Supporters of this type of legislation point to the fact that children understand things differently than their older counterparts. For example, one study showed that children who watch more television are less likely to know which types of food were less healthy than others. Other studies point to an explanation for this through their findings that showed nutrition-related information in advertisements shown on television are frequently misleading at best or inaccurate at worst and that children do not possess the necessary critical thinking skills to question what they are being shown. Mello and her colleagues, however, concluded that the Federal Trade Commission (FTC) is less likely to limit information made available to people and tends to rely on the idea that people will choose for themselves what information to take and believe and what information should be questioned or rejected outright.

What has been enacted at the federal level are regulations regarding food labels. Studies have shown that people are more likely to trust nutrition labels more than nutrition information provided via advertising. How we use these labels though may not be entirely as some would like. Some studies have shown that people do use nutrition labels to make healthier food choices but they are not that likely to use these labels explicitly for weight-loss efforts. Additionally, many restaurants provide nutritional information for their dishes despite the fact that they are not currently required to do so. One of the things that must be on food labels is fat content including the types of fat included in the food. Currently consuming trans fats has been linked to coronary heart disease and according to Gostin the Institute of Medicine has declared that there is no safe amount of trans fat that can be consumed and furthermore that there is no health benefit to human beings. Despite these findings and various regulations designed to protect the population from negative effects of this substance, Gostin notes that there are some who see any governmental measure as paternalistic and intrusive.

Gostin notes that opponents of governmental involvement suggest that providing health-based information is one thing, but enacting regulations that limit or prohibit how foods are manufactured can interfere with free market competition and ultimately interferes with individuals to decide for themselves whether or not they want to consume something that is more or less healthy for them. Additionally, they see governmental involvement and ultimately legal intervention as a paternalistic approach (i.e., using laws to tell people what they should and should not do as a parent would) that would ultimately undermine personal responsibility. By telling people what they can and cannot eat for example, people may come to rely on doing what they are told to do rather than making the decision themselves. Gostin writes that critics of things like a junk food or fat tax see this as a paternalistic measure and that since poor people are more likely to consume foods of this type it is also considered to be an effort targeting those who can least afford it. Moreover, he states that critics question where the proverbial line will be drawn in terms of which foods should be taxed and which should not.

The general population seems to be in favor of governmental involvement to a point. Adults may not want to be told what to do thereby infringing on their personal autonomy but are more likely to be supportive of measures designed to protect children. Michelle Mello and her colleagues offered suggestions for how to design laws and other regulations that are likely to be accepted by people in an effort to prevent and eliminate obesity. They noted that people are more likely to support initiatives that focus on children and adolescents who are considered to be vulnerable populations and therefore in need of protection. State laws and initiatives that exist for the purpose of combating obesity need to be empirically evaluated to determine if they have had the desired effect which would be a reduction in rates of obesity. Because advertising to children is, to date, not regulated, these authors suggest that counter-advertising may be in order; that is, advertising designed to educate and encourage children and adolescents to make healthier choices. They also noted that a public awareness campaign regarding how the food industry and food environment contribute to obesity is important for allowing consumers to be better informed and ultimately allowing them to make more healthy food-related decisions.

Mello's group's final thought is that personal responsibility and freedom to choose are not as straightforward as they seem. They noted that the multitude of forces (e.g., advertising, food manufacturing) that affect food and food choices may very well interfere with our ability to make truly informed and unbiased choices. In support of this notion, Ruth Armstrong in her article entitled "Obesity, Law and Personal Responsibility" summarized the thoughts and ideas shared at a professional conference. She noted the idea that personal choices are not made in a vacuum and that personal responsibility is influenced by what is going on around each of us. Thus, when there are laws and regulations designed to prevent unhealthy choices then our personal decisions will be influenced by that. Conversely, if public policy ignores the negative influences of things like deceptive or misleading advertising or the ways foods are manufactured then our personal decisions will be influenced by this. We would be more likely to make less healthy choices since we are not receiving information and counter-information indicating that this type of advertising is wrong or unhealthy. Freedom of choice and personal responsibility rests on the notion that we have all of the information we need to make a fully informed choice and that this information is unbiased and accurate. Without this, does true freedom to choose really exist?

This chapter has examined issues related to personal choice and the degree to which the government should be involved in regulating goods and services that may be connected to obesity. Critics of government involvement warn that too much involvement may result in people relying on being told what to do rather than on critically thinking and making rational, healthy decisions on their own. Others suggest that if the government does not get involved then those who are the most vulnerable (i.e., children and adolescents) will make less healthy decisions since they do not have the cognitive capacity to engage in critical thinking.

CHAPTER 9

Applications of Health at Every Size®

The applications for the Health at Every Size® (HAES®) approach are potentially numerous (a review of what the HAES® approach is can be found in Chapter 5). Given the fact that there are a multitude of efforts in myriad settings attempting to implement effective ways of helping overweight and obese individuals lose weight, it is theoretically possible to apply the HAES® approach to most settings. Regardless of the setting, the HAES® approach would require a cultural and paradigm shift from the belief that being overweight or obese is automatically unhealthy and that any overweight or obese individual should lose weight no matter what to the idea that engaging in healthy behaviors regardless of one's body size will help to improve a person's overall health and that this will occur regardless of weight that may or may not be lost. This section will explore where the HAES® approach has been applied and settings in which it could be applied.

HAES in Clinical Health Care

Clinical health-care refers to direct care provided to patients with a particular need. Health-care is intended to be a generic term and encompasses any profession or setting that addresses someone's physical or psychological well-being. This would include professions such as physicians, nurse practitioners, psychologists, social workers, other licensed mental health-care providers, registered dieticians, occupational therapists, physical therapists, and so on. Although much of the research on issues related to body size and quality of care is focused on physical health, some research has been applied to other allied professions as well (e.g., mental health).

A review of previous sections of this book will reveal that the application of the HAES® approach in clinical health-care settings would likely be beneficial. Chief among the concerns in community-based health-care is a concept known as anti-fat bias. As was discussed in Chapter 4, some health-care providers have been found to have this bias, meaning that they believe overweight and particularly obese individuals should lose weight. Those who have this bias are also more likely to believe that being overweight or obese is entirely within a person's control and that such patients can and should lose weight. The anti-fat bias often extends beyond a disdain for larger bodies and affects how the persons themselves are viewed. A health-care provider with an anti-fat bias may also see his or her patient as lazy, unmotivated, and not as intelligent as the patient's thinner counterparts. This attitude among health-care providers has been found to lead to spending less time with obese patients, being less likely to provide education about health behaviors in general, focus more or exclusively on weight loss, and less likely to order diagnostic testing that a thinner person with the same symptoms would receive. The result of this is that patients with larger bodies are less likely to schedule follow-up visits, schedule preventative screening appointments, and may not seek out health-care services at all. Some have argued that the effect anti-fat bias can have on health-care itself is a factor in the link between obesity and high health-care costs. If patients are not properly diagnosed by health-care providers or if they do not seek medical care at all, then it is likely that these patients will develop more health-related issues that if unidentified and untreated can evolve into chronic, debilitating, and potentially deadly diseases.

Instituting the HAES® approach in a health-care setting would mean that providers would be more likely to refrain from too quickly (or automatically) assuming that being overweight or obese is the cause of their medical concerns. Since the HAES® approach advocates for people engaging in healthy behaviors rather than engaging in behaviors for the purpose of weight loss no matter what, providers that take the HAES® approach will be more likely to recommend and prescribe interventions that they would also recommend and prescribe to patients with smaller body sizes. For example, they may encourage all of their patients to regularly engage in moderate physical activity while ensuring they are properly fueling their body based on activity level and internal hunger cues. An HAES® provider would also then assess the symptoms presented by the patient not from the point of view that being overweight or obese is the cause, but in terms of what the symptoms likely represent. Moreover, interventions would reflect the diagnosed issue (e.g., diabetes, high blood pressure) and the same intervention would be implemented not based on body size but based on symptoms alone. Additionally, when a diagnosis is not possible, further testing would be recommended again based on symptoms rather than body size.

An HAES® approach in health-care settings would also extend to elements of health-care beyond direct treatment and prevention. The atmosphere of the clinic or office would also be assessed in terms of how comfortable (physically or psychologically) an overweight or obese patient would be. Are the waiting room and the examining rooms designed to accommodate larger body sizes? Are medical devices sized such that they can be used on any body size (e.g., blood pressure cuffs)? Is weight-related data collected in a way that respects the privacy of the patient? Is the front-office staff respectful and courteous to all patients?

Since all aspects of a community-based health-care facility have the potential of contributing to the overall comfort or discomfort of an overweight or obese patient, the HAES® approach would only be effectively applied if all aspects of the facility are evaluated from this perspective and all personnel are educated on the philosophy behind the HAES® approach. In order for this approach to be effective, those in positions of power or authority (e.g., clinic owner, head physician) would need to embody the HAES® approach and respectfully confront comments, behaviors, or attitudes that are antithetical to this approach.

HAES in K-12 Schools

Many schools (i.e., grades K-12) across the United States have adopted health-related report cards that involve weighing children, recording the weight, and sending that information home to the child's parents or guardians. Some of these report cards include an explanation of why the report is being sent home, the purpose of the report, and what parents or guardians should do with the information. Some report cards simply include the child's weight, what their BMI is, and what weight class that puts them in (e.g., overweight, obese). Regardless of whether or not a report card is sent home and what may be included on the report cards themselves, it is clear that for many schools children's weight is an area of focus. Additionally, it is likely that most schools are dealing with weight-related bullying that may come from classmates, teachers, on-site health-care providers, or other school personnel.

Adopting the HAES® approach in schools can certainly be applied in the health-related services of the school. Many schools have a school nurse and a school counselor. School nurses familiar with the HAES® approach

to healthy living can learn how to more effectively and supportively interact with students of all body shapes and sizes, but particularly those who
are overweight or obese. School nurses are, of course, interested in making sure their students are as healthy as possible and may be inclined to
encourage weight loss efforts in students who are heavier regardless of
whether or not they are experiencing health problems. Students who hear
that weight loss is what they need to do are likely to take a hit to their self-
esteem. Many of these students may have tried to lose weight multiple
times without long-term success (see Chapter 7 for a discussion on what
may constitute long-term weight loss). Thus, hearing the weight-loss recommendation again from the school nurse may result in that child feeling
worse about themselves since an intervention they have already tried and
failed at is being recommended to them again. They may internalize this
as a personal failure and believe it is their fault they haven't lost enough or
any weight. It is also possible that this child may not be seeking future medical assistance or advice for fear of hearing the weight loss recommendation again. Taking the HAES® approach is likely to feel more encouraging
and empowering to a child. If they are encouraged to engage in behaviors
designed to enhance their overall health, they may have a greater chance of
feeling a sense of efficacy and success. This experience may lead the child
to continue the healthier behaviors and potentially adding new behaviors
on their own or with further non-weight-based encouragement.

There continues to be contentious debate among health-care providers
about the connection between weight and health especially when it comes
to the health of children. There is a multitude of data connecting larger
body sizes to an array of medical issues that range from mild to severe (see
Chapter 7). There is also a growing body of research suggesting that it is
not body size per se that is the cause of these medical issues but the degree
to which a particular person's body displays signs of metabolic syndrome
(see Chapter 7 for an explanation of this syndrome). Others suggest that
it is only a matter of time before someone with an obese body displays
symptoms of this syndrome even if they previously showed no signs of the
syndrome. Regardless of this conflict in perspective, what is a bit clearer
is that when people feel badly about themselves they are less likely to take
care of themselves and children are among those who may be more vulnerable to issues of self-esteem. If a child is continuously told to do something at which they have been unsuccessful (e.g., lose weight), they will
likely feel badly about themselves which can affect their overall mental
and physical health. Therefore, even if a school health-care provider is
staunchly in favor of weight loss for health reasons, the HAES® approach

can help such a provider convey their concern for the child's health in a way that can be heard and in a way that may allow a child to more naturally take up healthier behaviors. The tricky part, of course, is that engaging in objectively healthy behaviors (i.e., feeding the body what it needs rather than restricting intake, and engaging in regular physical activity) is no guarantee of weight loss—at least not the kind of weight loss that may move someone out of the obese category. This, then, may prove challenging for the school health-care provider who believes that weight loss by any means is the only avenue to health.

In addition to providing effective health-care, another challenge that many schools face is bullying. Bullying can and does occur for many reasons including race/ethnicity, religious beliefs, sexual orientation, weight, and so on. Weight-related bullying may be tacitly approved by schools that have a formal anti-obesity program. While the focus of programs like this are on obesity as a health issue, the problem with such efforts is that obesity itself is not a behavior that can be stopped or changed. Being obese is inextricably tied to the person. Thus, anti-obesity campaigns can become anti-obese person campaigns very quickly. Students, teachers, and other school personnel may feel empowered to comment on the body size of students under the guise of wanting to help the obese student get healthy. Moreover, some at the school may take their comments a step further by actively shaming the overweight or obese student through name-calling, making animal noises at them, expressing disgust when the student is eating, and so on. Some may do these things out of a spirit of meanness whereas others may believe that shaming someone who is overweight or obese will motivate them to lose weight and they therefore believe that shaming the student is helping the student.

Regardless of the intent behind any one person's interactions with an overweight or obese student, the atmosphere of the school itself can help shape how students of various shapes and sizes are not only perceived but also treated. Like most institutions and organizations, the atmosphere or culture of any given school is typically influenced by the highest levels of authority and power. Thus, if an anti-bullying campaign is instituted and the superintendent, principle, teachers, or health-care providers tell jokes or make comments that are about weight and size (their own or someone else's), then the campaign will likely not have the intended effect: that is, students treating other students kindly and with respect. Any HAES® program implemented in a school setting must first involve ensuring that those with the highest levels of authority and power are not only familiar with but also buy into the principles of the HAES® approach.

HAES® IN COLLEGES AND UNIVERSITIES

Like K-12 schools, colleges and universities have ample opportunity for implementing the HAES® approach. Although having and promoting a culture of HAES® on a college or university campus would be ideal, it may be less important than at a school where students are a captive audience for the entire day. Whereas students in grades K-12 are generally contained in one building and there are ample opportunities to interact with the same people multiple times per day, students on a campus of higher education may only see some people once or up to a few times per week. Thus, these students are less likely to be subjected to institutionalized or sanctioned weight-related stigma. Of course, there are exceptions to that which will be addressed here.

Before delving into specific issues on college campuses related to weight, there are ways that the HAES® approach can be applied on college and university campuses. As is the case with most K-12 schools, colleges and universities have some kind of health center. Given the rates of over-weight and obesity among the adult population of the United States (see Chapter 3 for prevalence data), many of those seeking health-care services will fall into weight categories including overweight and above. If health-care providers on college and university campuses are like health-care providers in community settings (and there is no reason to think they are not), then it is possible that overweight and obese students will not seek out health-care services for fear of an anti-fat bias (see Chapter 4 for an overview of anti-fat bias and its effects within health-care settings). Such a bias can lead to lack of seeking needed health care, less time receiving health-care from providers, and recommending weight loss as treatment regardless of the patient's immediate concern. Like their community-based counterparts, health-care providers on college and university cam-puses need to ensure that all personnel from those who provide direct care to front-office staff help to ensure that all patients feel comfortable and welcomed regardless of their body size. Instituting the HAES® approach can help in that effort in same manner as discussed in the section on apply-ing the HAES® approach to clinical health-care.

In addition to direct-care situations, it is also possible to apply the HAES® approach via college courses. Some courses may include the HAES® component for those studying a health-care profession or have a course devoted entirely to this perspective as a method or approach to health-care itself. It is also possible to expose most students on any col-lege or university campus to the HAES® approach by including it as a sec-tion or module in a required general education course. General education courses often include a standalone course or a module within a course devoted to personal care and wellness. This would be a logical place to include HAES® as one way of encouraging students to take care of themselves and their bodies. One college developed a general education course with a focus on the HAES® approach. Researchers Lauren Humphrey, Dawn Clifford, and Michelle Neyman Morris measured students on intuitive eating, body esteem, anti-fat attitudes, and dieting behavior who were enrolled in their institution's HAES® course. They compared these students to those enrolled in another course focused on health in general but not the HAES® approach in particular, and a to another group of students that did not receive any formal health-related instruction. The measures were collected for all students prior to the start of the semester and again at the end. The researchers found that students enrolled in the HAES® focused course showed significant improvements in intuitive eating, how they felt about their bodies, a decrease in anti-fat attitudes, and a reduction in diet-related behaviors compared to students in the other two groups. They further concluded that their finding suggest that enrolling in a course like this can have beneficial effects on college students.

Of course, some colleges will have entire courses or modules as part of courses that include content that is antithetical to the HAES® approach and instead focuses on the importance of weight loss as the only means of bolstering the health of someone who is overweight or obese. Beyond this, some campuses have instituted a requirement for overweight or obese students to lose weight. As such, implementing the HAES® approach campus-wide or at least providing information about this approach to decision makers may prevent situations as were found at one university in Pennsylvania.

In 2006, Lincoln University, for the first time, required its incoming class of students to take a *Fitness for Life* class prior to graduation or they would not receive their degrees. The issue was that this class was not required of all students, it was only required of those with a BMI over 30 (i.e., obese). Some health experts indicated that the university's concern for their students' health was admirable while others noted that when health standards are imposed on people they struggle to meet them. Additionally, some pointed to the now more widely understood flaw of using BMI as an indicator or health or obesity (see Chapter 2 for a discussion of BMI) since highly muscular individuals may be classified as obese due to the density of muscle mass which contributes to one's overall weight. Regardless of the intent of this measure, the article describing Lincoln University's efforts points out that it may have backfired since students who were required to take the course due to their BMI were singled out as being unhealthy and obese. Some students noted that focusing on the health and well-being of students should mean that no body shape or size should be singled out; rather, all students should be encouraged (or required) to improve their overall health and fitness.

Whether a college or university has formal plans to address the overall wellness of their students or not, there are myriad ways the HAES® approach can be applied within this setting from the health-care office to college courses.

HAES AND PUBLIC HEALTH-CARE POLICY

It could be argued that applying the HAES® approach to public health-care policy is desperately needed since much effort has been focused in recent years on the obesity epidemic and the subsequent war on obesity. Of course, given the fact that not all health-care providers or health-care policy makers agree on whether or not being overweight or obese is inherently bad for one's health, the approach taken has been to stay the course and treat obesity as something to be eliminate because it is a disease in and of itself.

The HAES® approach could most certainly be applied to health-care policy decisions; however, doing so would require including this approach at the highest levels of government—local, state, or federal. Currently, the prevailing attitude is that obesity is the most significant modern health crisis. Many national health-care-related organizations have position statements addressing how their professionals can help treat obesity. Former First Lady, Michelle Obama, developed her *Let's Move!* campaign for the express purpose of combating obesity among children. The HAES® approach would applaud the first lady's efforts at encouraging children to engage in healthy behaviors, but would suggest that all children would benefit from this message because no one can tell who is healthy and who is not simply by looking their body weight, shape, or size.

Policies designed for the purpose of addressing obesity, particularly among children, have included things like BMI report cards, zoning regulations with regards to how many fast food restaurants can exist in an area, and regulations around what kinds of foods and how much food is served in school cafeterias and vending machines. Some of the policies are likely beneficial regardless of the reason for their implementation, however, policies such as BMI report cards have been shown to have negative effects on children and may, in some cases, lead to the development of eating disorders. Another potential issue for these policies is outcome. If the purpose of implementing these policies is to reduce childhood obesity, what happens if obesity rates do not decline or the children affected by the policies show no meaningful change in weight? Are the policies abandoned even if they promote healthy behaviors? Removing the focus on weight can help make clear which policies will benefit people regardless of what they weigh. The HAES® approach applied to health-care policy could help make that happen.

If policy makers used the HAES® approach for drafting health-care-related programs, they would be much more likely to have the health of all citizens in mind rather than targeting those who, in this case, have a body size that is larger than what many people believe is healthy. Removing the connection between weight and health will ensure that health-related policies make recommendations based on health from which all citizens can benefit. Additionally, in order to determine the effectiveness of such policies physicians can rely on objective measures of health such as blood pressure, blood sugar, degree of inflammation, and so on, rather than relying on the number on a scale or BMI.

Relying on weight can result in assuming an overweight or obese person is unhealthy when they are not, and assuming a normal or even underweight person is healthy when they are not. When this occurs, health-care-related policies narrowly applied (e.g., to obese individuals only) end up helping those who do not need it, and missing those who are in desperate need of the message.

HAES in the Workplace

There are many aspects of the work environment on which the HAES® approach can be applied, not the least of which are wellness programs. Many workplaces have wellness programs that include things like access to gyms, swimming pools, health screenings, flu shots, and so on. The purpose of these programs is to promote overall health and well-being among employees. This is a good thing for companies as employers will benefit from a healthier workforce who will miss fewer days of work, be more productive overall, and will have lower health insurance premiums. Because one's weight is believed by many to be a strong indicator of one's overall health, it is not surprising that many companies use weight-based and weight-loss incentive programs for their employees. Some of these incentives may come in the form of paying less for health insurance and other incentives may take the form of gift cards or other prizes for those who lose the most weight over some period of time. The assumption, of course, is that if weight is being lost then the person is getting healthier; however, there is usually no mechanism in place for determining what each employee may be doing to lose that weight, whether their health has actually benefitted from their weight loss, whether or not weight loss was healthy for them to do in the first place, or if those who haven't lost any weight are healthier as a result of engaging in healthier behaviors.

Using the HAES® approach in the context of employee wellness programs would decidedly take the focus off weight and turn it more directly to objective measures of health. Instead of having weight loss competitions, healthier behavior-based competitions may be more effective in promoting overall health. Given the technology that exists in this day and age, it is relatively easy to track activity levels and types of foods eaten on a daily or weekly basis. Implementing competitions based on healthy behaviors or encouraging employees to simply track their health-related behaviors can send the message that the employer is interested in the overall health of their employees rather than what size their bodies are.

In many ways a workplace is a microcosm of the larger society. As such many of the issues discussed in previous sections of this chapter can be applied to the workplace. For example, a company that promotes the HAES® perspective would be more sensitive to the needs of a wide range of body weights, shapes, and sizes and would ensure that work spaces comfortably accommodate all body sizes. Facilities such as restrooms and lunch areas, too, would be designed with a range of body sizes in mind. The overall atmosphere of a workplace with the HAES® perspective as part of its culture will feel better to those who often feel ostracized, shamed, or in other ways oppressed simply because of the size of their body. This would not be tolerated at a workplace with the HAES® approach and would likely be met with the recognition that there is an ongoing need to educate their employees about harassment in general and the HAES® in particular to ensure that the work environment feels safe for everyone.

HAES® IN FITNESS-RELATED VENUES

Fitness-related venues include locations such as gyms, the YMCA, physical therapy practices, and anywhere where there is a focus on exercise, fitness, and/or nutrition. Given the focus on fitness in these facilities, it is not surprising that people who do not already fit the ideal body type for either males or females may feel intimidated or even unwelcomed at these places. In fact, it is possible for someone to be publically shamed for their body as illustrated by numerous examples of people taking photos of overweight or obese individuals working out and then commenting derisively on their bodies. One of the more well-known examples of this was in 2016 when Dani Mathers, a Playboy Playmate, took picture of a naked woman who was going about her business in the locker room. Dani posted the photo via Snapchat with the caption "If I can't unsee this then you can't either." She was inundated by internet comments condemning her actions and calling what she did a criminal act. Ms. Mathers lost her membership at that gym and apparently lost her job as well. She was subsequently criminally charged with invasion of privacy.

Certainly, the actions of any individual are beyond the control of any facility; however, when the focus of any fitness-related intervention is on weight loss or weight maintenance the message is clear: how much you weigh is the most important factor. The implication of a weight-based focus in fitness-related venues is that being a certain weight or size will lead to being fit and healthy. Additionally, when the message is weight loss for those who are overweight or obese (and even those who are considered to be normal weight), these patrons are likely to feel singled out and that there is something wrong with them that requires fixing. This can create an attitude of disgust for one's body and make it much more difficult to be motivated to take care of it. Additionally, when the motive to exercise is to lose weight what happens when the weight is lost? Is more weight loss desired? Is there no other reason to continue to work out? When taking care of one's body and improving one's overall health is the goal, it becomes easier to see why ongoing exercise is important. Moreover, a focus on how one feels as their body becomes more fit rather than on the number on a scale is likely to be more rewarding in the long term. Focusing on experiences such as these would be consistent with the HAES® approach.

At venues where the focus is on fitness and health, there is ample opportunity to incorporate the philosophy and teachings of the HAES® approach. Educating staff on the HAES® approach from those working the reception desk to personal trainers leading classes or working one-on-one with clients can help to create a climate not only of acceptance of all body types but also of supporting the efforts of all patrons, regardless of body size, who invest in becoming more fit and healthier. Applying the HAES® approach to personnel who work at a fitness-related venue will help them encourage and motivate patrons based on how they feel both physically and psychologically rather than continuously reminding them that their sole purpose for sweating is to shed unwanted pounds or eliminate love handles.

HAES® IN PUBLIC SERVICES

Public services in this section refer to any business that provides a service directly to consumers. This might include things like restaurants, public transportation, hair dressers, or airlines. A great deal of attention has been paid to airlines and how they accommodate, or do not accommodate, larger sized bodies (see Chapter 4 for a more detailed discussion on obesity and airlines). Debate has involved who should pay when some bodies require more space than smaller bodies, and what should happen when someone with a smaller body feels like their space is infringed upon by sitting next to someone occupying a seat that is not built to accommodate their size? Regardless of the setting or service provided, generally speaking these companies are not in the business of facilitating consumer's health. They are merely providing a service that is needed or desired but not necessarily health-related. Despite this, the HAES® perspective can be usefully applied to the service industry as well.

One of the benefits of learning about and applying the HAES® approach is the shift in thinking that can occur when HAES® principles are internalized. The HAES® approach reminds people that engaging in healthy behaviors regardless of size will enhance the person's overall health. They may or may not lose any weight; however, when weight is no longer the focus and the focus shifts to healthy behaviors, then it may become more possible to accept people as they are no matter their body shape or size. As examined in Chapter 4, how people with larger bodies are treated by the airlines and airline passengers reveals that many people have the perspective that people with larger bodies are a nuisance and a hindrance to others' comfort. An underlying implication is that if only they would do something about it (i.e., lose weight) then there would not be a problem. A further assumption made by someone with this perspective is that someone's weight is entirely within their control. As discussed in Chapter 7, there are a multitude of factors at play that affect the weight, size, and shape of our bodies, many of which are beyond any one individual's control.

Public services that take on the HAES® philosophy are more likely to recognize that their customers come in a variety of shapes and sizes and that it would benefit all of the consumers to accommodate all sizes rather than only serving or accommodating the average body size. Employees of services that incorporate the HAES® approach will also be more likely to treat their larger bodied customers with the respect deserved by all customers. Thus, they will be less likely to see someone who is lazy or unmotivated, but as a human being who happens to have a larger body and is seeking a service just like everyone else.

The HAES® approach is a philosophy that takes the focus off body weight, shape, and size and redirects it to health in general. There are myriad settings in which the HAES® approach can be applied and the most obvious settings are those that have an explicit focus on health. Other settings, however, can benefit from this approach as well. Although such businesses provide services that do not necessarily directly affect health their approach to their patrons can indirectly affect the health of those with larger bodies by showing acceptance regardless of their body size and by having settings that easily and readily accommodate any body size.

PART III

Scenarios

CHAPTER 10

Case Illustrations

In this section, five different scenarios will be presented depicting someone actively struggling with their weight, being told that they should be concerned about their weight, and/or someone considering options for weight loss. Each scenario will be described and then followed by an analysis from the mainstream perspective (i.e., how most people and healthcare providers typically approach weight and health) and from the Health at Every Size® (HAES®) perspective.

Scenario 1: Karl Receives a BMI Report Card from School

Karl is eight years old and in third grade. His school, like many across the United States, has adopted a plan to focus on the health of children by identifying those who are overweight or obese and informing the parents of these children via a BMI or fitness report card. Each child in Karl's school was weighed as part of a regularly scheduled physical education class. Each child's weight was recorded on a form that indicated if the child was underweight, normal weight, overweight, or obese. The form with this information was sent home to the child's parents along with instructions for the parents to consult with their child's physician regarding their child's weight. The intent behind these report cards is to ensure that parents are informed about their child's health as it relates to their weight and to encourage the parents along with the child to take action to reduce the child's weight if he or she is overweight or obese.

Karl came home from school the day he was weighed and according to his mother seemed out of sorts. He was angry, threw his backpack on the ground, and slammed doors. When his mother inquired what was wrong, he said, "Nothing. I'm just fat and everybody knows it." When she asked why he thought this, Karl rifled through his backpack to find the BMI report card and slapped it on the kitchen counter.

Karl's mom read the form and looked at the graph indicating where Karl's BMI fell on the BMI percentile chart. The chart was color-coded: green for normal weight, yellow for overweight, and red for obese. There was also a pink category on the opposite end of the scale for those who were underweight. In the red section was an "X" to indicate this was the category in which Karl's weight fell. Karl's mom read the explanation for this category which stated that Karl was classified as obese and that they should schedule an appointment with his pediatrician as soon as possible to discuss a plan for reducing Karl's weight. There were also pointers for encouraging healthy eating and increasing physical activity.

Karl's mother scheduled an appointment with his pediatrician within two weeks. At the appointment Karl's mother showed the physician the BMI report card. She immediately expressed concern about Karl's health but added that she wasn't sure what she could do to help him lose weight because she noted that he already eats fairly healthy (several servings of fruits and vegetables per day) along with lean meats, and that he participates in a sport nearly year round. The physician too expressed concern about Karl's weight and his overall health indicating that because he is obese he is at greater risk for developing serious health problems which may interfere with daily functioning at best and may cause an early death at worst. The physician prescribed a reduction in caloric intake and an increase in physical activity. He scheduled a follow-up visit for three months later and said that he expected meaningful weight loss by the next appointment.

Analysis

Clearly all those involved with Karl are concerned about his health and want what is best for him. The pediatrician's recommendations are in-line with conventional thinking about weight and health. A child with a BMI that places them in the obese category will be met with a fervent attitude of weight loss quickly so that they have a chance to be healthy now and stave off the development of diseases known to be linked to obesity. In this situation, Karl's mother expressed concern that her son already eats well and is regularly physically active. At this point, it would be useful for the physician to inquire more about Karl's eating and physical activity habits. It is certainly possible that Karl is not engaged in entirely healthy behaviors (or not as healthy as the mom thinks) and has room for improvement. There were no specifics given with respect to the amount of caloric reduction expected, the degree of increase in physical activity expected, or the amount of weight loss. It is therefore possible that Karl's parents may do whatever is necessary to have Karl show meaningful weight loss by the next scheduled appointment.

The HAES® approach to this scenario would likely be different. A pediatrician familiar with and invested in the HAES® approach would have certainly gotten Karl's height and weight and compared his current stats to his previous stats on his growth chart (see Chapter 2 to read more about growth carts). A dramatic change in percentile with respect to height or weight might indicate an area of concern. Apart from that, however, the pediatrician taking the HAES® approach would gather standard checkup data and talk with both Karl and his mother about the degree to which he is physically active as well as his typical eating habits. The pediatrician would also likely ask if there is room for improvement in healthy behaviors—which the HAES® pediatrician would ask of any child regardless of BMI. Taking this approach with Karl emphasizes Karl's overall health as measured by standard assessments and comparing the information gathered with standard health markers as well as Karl's own health history. A pediatrician taking this approach may also ask Karl and/or his mother if they have concerns about his body size knowing that most people do. If they did have concerns, the pediatrician would educate them both on the HEAS® approach and the emphasis on encouraging healthy behaviors, continuing to monitor Karl's overall health as would be done with any child, and making recommendations based on assessment data rather than on weight itself.

As noted at the beginning of this analysis, the approach taken by the pediatrician in the scenario is consistent with standard practice when a child has a BMI in the obese range. Parents of children like Karl who receive a recommendation for their child to lose weight could consult with a dietician specializing in pediatric nutrition to ensure that he continues to get nutritionally what his body needs as they pursue weight loss and potentially increase the child's physical activity. Alternatively, the parents could learn more about the HAES® approach, talk with their pediatrician about his or her willingness to work with their child from this perspective, and potentially change pediatricians if they are unwilling to do so.

Scenario 2: Sarah Wants to Gain Weight to Be More Curvy

Sarah is an 18-year-old young woman who is finishing her senior year of high school and preparing to go to college. She has not dated very much throughout her adolescence and has frequently overheard some of her peers (both males and females) refer to her as scrawny and say things like she "doesn't have much meat on her bones." Growing up she was identified as overweight but when she grew two inches one summer all of the weight she had seemed to be used up making her taller. She always thought skinnier was better and more attractive but now that she was developing as a young woman she thought she'd be curvier. When she looks at herself in the mirror she sees the body of a prepubescent girl rather than a woman. She knows that she is post puberty as she has been menstruating since she was 12, and her breasts did grow some but compared to most of her female classmates she had nothing on her chest, and padded or push-up bras did not help much.

Sarah was envious of her female classmates who seemed to be able to just walk into the room and have all eyes on them. She wished she could look like the underwear models she saw on the annual lingerie runway show on TV. They were, by conventional standards, thin but most definitely had breasts that filled up bra sizes much larger than hers and their bare midriffs highlighted the fact that their waists were much smaller than their hips which contributed to the hourglass look she longed for.

Sarah had always valued her health and well-being. As a result she ate well, never skimped on calories or types of food but focused on fruits, vegetables, and lean meats, and she engaged in regular exercise by jogging most days of the week. Although she physically felt well and had all the energy she needed to stay focused on her course work and run around with her dog after school, she did not feel emotionally well. She hated her body and regularly thought of herself as ugly since no one wanted to date her. Her friends told her not to worry about it and that anyone worth anything would not care about how she looked but who she was on the inside. Sarah usually appreciated her friends' attempt at support but she often felt like they didn't get it.

Sarah decided her only course of action would be to gain weight. She planned to reduce how much exercise she engaged in and increase the amount of high calorie, high fat foods she ate. She followed her new plan for a month and saw the scale continue to rise as planned; however, she noticed that although her breasts were growing larger so was her stomach, arms, and legs. She realized she was getting fat and now overheard some of her peers saying things like she was getting chubby. One time a female classmate yelled down the hall at her "Hey Sarah! A moment on the lips, a lifetime on the hips! You need to lose weight girl!" Dejected, Sarah resolved to go on a diet and lose weight not matter what.

Analysis

It is unclear from this scenario if Sarah would be considered overweight at this point or where she would have fallen on the BMI chart to begin with. What is clear, however, is that Sarah has struggled to be happy with her body no matter what weight she has been. Sarah's desire to first gain weight to try to look more like the curvy runway models and classmates she has envied, and then to lose weight because she was gaining weight all over rather than in only areas that would make her curvier puts her at risk for yo-yo dieting. Although this has not yet become a pattern for Sarah, her dissatisfaction at any weight thus far as an adult and her longing to be perceived as attractive to her peers suggests she could fall into this unhealthy pattern.

A conventional approach to Sarah's concern about her weight would be to determine her ideal weight based on BMI (see Chapter 2 for more on BMI) and offer recommendations for her to get to and stay in her ideal weight range based on her age and height. Depending on how far away she is, and on which side of her ideal BMI she is, Sarah may receive recommendations to either gain weight or lose weight. If she needs to lose weight she might also be encouraged to engage in exercise or intensify what she is already doing. If she needs to gain weight she may be encouraged to cut back on her physical activity. It is possible that an assessment for an eating disorder is warranted. Although there is not enough information from this scenario to determine whether or not this is a concern, someone who focuses heavily on their weight and appearance may be at greater risk for developing an eating disorder. This can be a concern even if Sarah's weight is *within the normal range on the BMI chart*. She may also receive a referral to a mental health professional to help her with self-esteem related concerns.

The HAES® approach would encourage Sarah to focus on her health and allow her body to be whatever weight, shape, and size, it will be given healthy eating and healthy exercise behaviors. She would be encouraged to eat a wide range of foods that she enjoys eating and identifying physical activity or exercise that she also enjoys. If she is not sure how to eat healthy (especially if she has gotten into a pattern of yo-yo dieting), she may receive a referral to a registered dietician who can help ensure her body is getting what it needs. Should Sarah continue to struggle with accepting her body as it is, she may receive a referral to a licensed mental health professional who may work with her on issues such as self-esteem and body acceptance. Depending on how Sarah talks about herself, her body, food, exercise, and weight, she may also benefit from an assessment for an eating disorder. Identifying an eating disorder as soon as possible will be important for Sarah's overall physical and emotional health.

SCENARIO 3: GEORGE IS CONSIDERING WEIGHT-LOSS SURGERY

George is a 45-year-old man who is married and has two children. He feels like he has everything going for him since he likes his job, has a good marriage, and his children are happy and healthy. However, George has struggled with his weight for most of his life. He seemed to have solved his weight problem during high school when he went through puberty and became a three-sport athlete. He could eat anything he wanted and never gained weight. He played two sports at a Division II university in his first two years of college but then decided to devote his time and energy to becoming a lawyer. He knew he needed excellent grades to get into law school and to prepare well for the law school entrance exam. He noticed that he gained some weight during those last two years of college before entering law school but attributed that to stress and not eating very well. He knew he was not as active as he had been, but figured if he was only going to gain ten pounds or so he could live with that.

As the years went on and his overall stress level increased with law school, then becoming a lawyer, and establishing himself in his profession; he continued to gain weight. He found that he was not only the heaviest he had ever been but that he did not seem to have the strength he once had and was easily winded walking up stairs. He decided he needed to do something about it so he went on a self-designed diet. He reduced the amount of calories he ate by half and cut out foods with fat, foods with added sugar, and most forms of bread. He also resumed physical activity by going for a long walk at least three days a week. He noticed a change in his weight and energy level within two weeks and was motivated to continue; however, after another two weeks he noticed his energy level drop which he attributed to increased stress at work. He had to take on more clients when one of his colleagues left unexpectedly. This also left less time for going for walks or working out in any other way. As a result, his weight climbed again and exceeded the weight at which he started prior to his diet.

The following 15 years involved George going on and off diets, and starting and stopping various exercise routines. Some of what he did was self-designed, and some involved formal programs that he paid for. George estimates he has been on a diet on at least 20 different occasions and knows he has spent thousands of dollars on gym memberships, diet foods, weight-loss programs, and personal coaching. Despite all of the time, effort, and money he has poured into losing weight, George's weight is at the highest it has ever been. He weighs 70 pounds more than when he started his first diet. George has researched bariatric surgery (a.k.a. weight-loss surgery; see Chapter 3 for more information on weight-loss surgery) and knows that he would qualify for most procedures based on his weight alone; his BMI is currently 38 (class II obesity; see Chapter 2 for more information on BMI). He is currently scheduled for a pre-weight loss surgery assessment and hopes to have his surgery scheduled within a month. He is looking forward to finally being thin again and being able to stay that way.

Analysis

George has clearly been stuck in a pattern of yo-yo dieting for many years, which is a common experience of many people whose weight initially climbs higher than what is deemed to be attractive or ideal in terms of health. Also, like many people who have gone on and off diets, George's weight is higher than when he first started dieting. Research has shown that this is an expected outcome of yo-yo dieting and some research has found that going on a diet even one time can predict weight gain rather than weight loss. Given George's frustration with his body, and presumably with himself for not being able to lose weight and keep it off, he has decided to pursue weight loss surgery anticipating that the surgery will finally allow him to lose and keep the weight off for good.

Prior to George getting this surgery, he will need to complete a pre-surgery assessment which is standard practice with weight loss surgeries. The purpose of the assessment is to measure the surgical patient's goals for the surgery, their understanding of what the surgery can and cannot do, and any history of medical or psychological issues that may affect success with the surgery (e.g., an eating disorder diagnosis). George should also be counseled with respect to not only what will be involved with the surgery which can include having part of his stomach or intestines removed, having his intestines rerouted, or making only a small portion of his stomach available for food. He will also be counseled on how he must change his eating habits immediately after surgery, and what he will need to do for the rest of his life to maintain his overall health. Finally, George should be counseled with regard to possible results of the surgery, which can include infection, bleeding, hernia, not losing as much weight as expected, regaining of some or all of the weight lost, and in some cases complications that lead to death. Should George decide that he does not want to pursue weight loss surgery or is not a candidate for the surgery it may be recommended that George try a weight loss medication that can have side effects George may find unpleasant and none are intended for long-term use.

An alternative to weight loss by any means is the HAES® approach, which would redirect George's focus toward health and away from weight. He would be encouraged to engage in healthy behaviors which included eating a variety of foods that he enjoys and also provide the nutrients his body needs, and would include engaging in regular physical activity or exercise that he finds enjoyable, especially whatever he can easily work into the course of his day. Part of this approach would certainly involve weight loss from the perspective that he may or may not lose weight based on adopting and maintaining healthy eating and activity habits but that his body will be the shape and size it needs to be once it is regularly and properly fed and moved around. He would need to know too that a history of yo-yo dieting may have permanently changed how his body metabolizes food which will mean that weight loss regardless of behaviors will be quite difficult. Encouraging a focus on health and healthy behaviors, however, will allow George to focus on how he feels physically and psychologically, as he takes care of his body and lets go of the focus on weight loss.

SCENARIO 4: MAYA'S DOCTOR TOLD HER TO LOSE WEIGHT

Maya is a 29-year-old woman who is married and planning to have a family in the next few years. She recently had her annual physical exam which revealed that she is in excellent health—as she has been her entire life. Her blood work indicated that the ratio between her low-density lipoprotein cholesterol (aka good cholesterol) and her high-density lipoprotein cholesterol (aka bad cholesterol) is low, which suggests that she is at low risk for heart disease. Additionally, her blood pressure is well within the normal range, and other indicators of health status such as glucose (i.e., blood sugar), triglycerides, and complete blood count all indicate that she is in very good health.

Maya smiles when she hears the results and says to her doctor, "I'm not too surprised. Most of my family is healthy and live well beyond the average life span. And besides, I take good care of myself. I eat healthy, get enough sleep, and work out a lot so I can stay in shape for my weekend soccer league. We play indoors during the winter." She expected to receive a proverbial pat on the back from her doctor but when Maya looked at her, her doctor had a concerned look on her face. Maya asked what was wrong and wondered if there was some other test that showed she had some kind of serious disease that simply wasn't affecting how she felt yet.

Her doctor said, "Yes all of that is really good, but I'm concerned about your weight. Last time we met you were on the high end of the overweight range. Since then you've gained a few pounds and now you are officially obese which puts you at significant risk for all kinds of serious diseases like diabetes, cardiovascular disease, stroke, and some forms of cancer. It is really important that we talk about how you are going to lose weight."

Maya said she was confused because all the tests that the doctor ordered clearly showed that she was healthy and that there were no results that indicated there could be a problem. Maya asked, "Aren't these results the same as they were last year and all of the years before that? Nothing has gotten worse has it?" Her doctor agreed that the tests showed and have historically showed that she has been in good health, but that it was simply a matter of time before these results change and her body starts to show signs of problems. The doctor handed Maya a sheet with recommended weight loss tips the first of which suggested that she decrease how much she ate and increase how much she exercised. She also received the name of a registered dietitian who would "help you tweak your diet so it is healthier."

Maya left the appointment confused and concerned. She wondered how much time she had before a serious problem showed up, but was confused because she wasn't sure how she could eat any healthier than she already was—she had previously worked with a dietitian to craft a diet that fueled her body based on the amount of activity she engaged in and that was nutrient dense. She also didn't know how much more physical activity she could do. She already went to the gym three times a week, practiced with her team two times a week, and played two games on the weekend. She was worried that doing any more might result in injury. Nonetheless, she trusted that her doctor must know more than she does, and she scheduled an appointment with the new dietitian with the goal of figuring out how to lose weight. She worried that the only remedy left was to cut overall calories and that she would be hungry all of the time.

Analysis

Maya's physician's recommendations are in line with what many if not most physicians would recommend. It is common medical practice for someone who is significantly overweight or obese is to recommend weight loss regardless of other measures that reveal there are no areas of concern. A great deal of research has linked obesity specifically to several serious diseases including cardiovascular disease, some forms of cancer, diabetes, sleep problems, and osteoarthritis (see Chapter 6 for a discussion of this research). Many researchers have concluded that weight loss is necessary to prevent such diseases from developing even when there are no indicators that a particular person is at risk for those diseases. Some research has also shown that when weight loss occurs in those who have a particular diagnosis connected with obesity their symptoms improve or go away altogether.

Other researchers have challenged these findings by looking at underlying mechanisms that may explain both obesity and associated diseases, and by examining underlying processes that may explain the improvement of symptoms with weight loss. Recent research, for example, has found that something called the metabolic syndrome (see Chapter 7 for a discussion of this syndrome) is a constellation of symptoms that is linked to the diseases associated with obesity and that these symptoms (and accompanying diseases) are not found among all who are obese. Moreover, these symptoms can be found in as many as 30 percent of those who are normal weight. There are also those pointing to the idea that even if weight loss might show improvement in symptoms—though not all research shows this—there are those who indicate that long-term weight loss (i.e., weight loss that is maintained for at least five years) is not reliably possible (see Chapter 7 for a discussion of weight loss research).

The HAES® approach suggests that weight loss in and of itself, regardless of whether or not it is possible to achieve long term, is not a goal that will lead to overall health. Those who take this approach would recommend to Maya that she should not change what she is doing since she routinely engages in healthy eating and regularly engages in physical activity. Moreover, because there are no signs that there is any medical issue based on standard medical tests, there is no reason for her to make any changes. She is adequately fueling her body (which was confirmed by a registered dietician prior to her medical visit) and giving it reasonable exercise, and her body is the weight and size it needs to be. Those who take the HAES® approach point to the idea that not all bodies can be in the normal weight range on a BMI chart and be healthy; healthy bodies come in all shapes and sizes. The important thing is to be sure Maya continues to engage in healthy behaviors to support what her healthy body is currently capable of doing.

Scenario 5: Samantha Has Decided to Stop Dieting and Focus on Health

Samantha is a 24-year-old woman who has been on and off diets most of her life. As a child she was considered chunky and was often made fun of by her peers because of her weight. She was also regularly encouraged to watch what she was eating by her mother and older sister, and when she had her annual doctor's checkup Samantha was routinely found to be healthy with basic standard measures of health; however, her mother was encouraged by the pediatrician to put Samantha on a diet to get her to a healthier weight. Her mother initially restricted the amount of food Samantha was allowed to eat, and then gradually started to limit the types of foods she could eat. Samantha was hungry most of the time and learned early on to not ask for more food because her mother consistently told her no and that she had "had enough." As Samantha grew older and had more control over what and how much she ate, she continued to experiment with diets based on what her classmates had tried and what she read about in magazines and online. She knew that being thinner was something she should strive to be regardless of how hungry she was or how low her energy levels became.

When Samantha began a new diet and started to lose weight, her friends, family, and acquaintances would notice and praise her for her efforts. She also realized that more men seemed to find her attractive and that her female peers often asked her what her secret was so they could lose weight too. When she regained the weight after no longer being able to continue a diet she was met with sympathy and support but inside she felt like she was a failure as a person. On nearly every diet she tried, as a child, adolescent, and now young adult Samantha initially lost weight. The most she ever lost on one diet was 30 pounds and the least was five pounds. She was never, however, able to keep the weight off because she was never able to sustain the diets themselves. As a result she always regained what she had lost and over the last several years realized that her overall weight had continued to rise and was currently 10 pounds more than what she had weighed at the end of high school. Every time Samantha regained the weight she had lost on a diet she felt like a failure and that it was her lack of willpower that made her fail at dieting. Prior to beginning a new diet she resolved for herself that this time her willpower would be stronger and she would be able to keep going with the diet. She had not sustained any diet for more than one year.

On her most recent birthday Samantha ceremoniously blew out the candles on her birthday cake and wished for the willpower to begin and sustain a diet that would finally keep the weight off forever. She felt good about her wish until she thought about it some more and wondered why this time would be any different than all of the times before. She could not come up with any answer. She then wondered what it might be like for her to stop dieting, stop trying to lose weight, and simply try to live as healthy a life as possible. She began reading as much as she could about what were considered to be healthy behaviors while avoiding articles and books with weight loss as a focus or even a by-product.

Analysis

It is unclear from this scenario what BMI classification Samantha was as a child or what she is now. If she is in the overweight or one of the obese categories she will likely receive the recommendation by her primary-care provider at her annual checkup that she should lose weight. If they discuss Samantha's diet and weight-loss history she will probably still receive the weight-loss recommendation and may receive referrals to a registered dietician, weight-loss support groups, and other services designed to help people lose weight and keep it off. It is likely, given Samantha's current perspective on dieting and weight loss that she will not follow up on these recommendations. She may seek out a new primary-care provider who is supportive of engaging in healthy behaviors while still monitoring her overall health to be sure her body continues to function as it should. Should Samantha look for a new primary-care provider who can provide this type of care for her she would likely be drawn to someone who follows the HAES® approach.

A provider taking the HAES® approach with Samantha would support her decision to discard dieting and weight loss as a goal along with shifting her focus toward healthy behaviors. She would be encouraged to meet with a registered dietician, if needed, to help her identify foods she enjoys eating but that provide her body nutritionally what it needs. She would also be encouraged to engage in physical activity that she enjoys, and to experiment with various activities until she finds what works for her.

Samantha may be met with concern by family, friends, and other health-care providers when they learn that she is no longer trying to lose weight so she is in the normal weight BMI category. They will probably encourage her to not diet if that is not what she wants to do but to change her lifestyle. Their recommendations, however, will likely include things like cutting back on calories, cutting out or heavily reducing sugar, fat and simple carbohydrates, and intensifying her exercise routine. Samantha may or may not choose to respond to these recommendations outwardly;

however, she is likely to be aware of the fact that these recommendations are exactly what she has tried previously—none of which worked for her in terms of long-term weight loss.

Samantha may struggle with wondering if it truly is her willpower that is at issue, and if she only tried harder she would lose weight and keep it off. In her readings she will have come across research indicating that there may be things she can and should do differently so she can achieve long-term weight loss. She will also, however, read about studies indicating that achieving a particular weight is not a matter of willpower but is function of the complex interaction between genetics, behaviors, and environmental factors (e.g., how food is manufactured and advertised). The HAES® approach would remind her that when she takes care of her body though regular physical activity and eating in a healthy but enjoyable way her body will be whatever shape and size it needs to be in order to be healthy. This may mean she does not fit into the normal range of the BMI scale.

GLOSSARY

Anti-Fat Bias: Anti-fat bias refers to a negative attitude someone has about large, usually obese bodies. When someone has this bias it has been found that not only is there a negative view of an obese person's body but also of that person as a human being (e.g., they are lazy, unmotivated, not smart).

Bariatric Surgery: Also known as weight loss surgery, bariatric surgery refers to a number of different surgical procedures designed to alter the digestive system to prevent weight gain and promote weight loss.

BMI Report Cards: A BMI report card is a report sent home to parents of children enrolled in K-12 schools. The report includes the child's body mass index (BMI) along with its classification (e.g., normal weight, obese). Some reports include recommendations of what to do with this information. Not all schools distribute such reports.

Body Mass Index (BMI): BMI is a mathematical formula that divides a person's weight in kilograms by their height in meters squared. The equation was developed in 1832 by Adolphe Quetelet who was attempting to determine what constituted the average man.

Comstock Law: A law passed in 1873 that prohibited the distribution of material referring to sex or the sexuality of women which at the time include materials about birth control.

Fashion Plate: A term referring to an individual wearing the popular fashions of the day. The term is derived from the practice of printing these images in magazines by using hand-colored engravings.

Flapper: The moniker for the 1920s' modern woman. She was young, usually mid-teens to mid-twenties. Her wardrobe revealed her neck and throat, and her skirt fell just below her knees—the outfit did not hug her curves. Flappers had short stylized hair and were generally flat chested.

Focusing Illusion: The focusing illusion is a psychological concept that refers to our tendency to focus on one thing in our lives that we either have (or have experienced) or do not have (or have not experienced), and assume that if the thing or event is good then we will be happier and if the thing or event is bad then we will suffer. The illusion refers to the idea that our assumptions about what will happen as a result of positive or negative experiences are false.

Gibson Girl: Charles Gibson was an artist who created print images of both males and females wearing the latest fashions of the late 1900s. His portrayal of women (commonly referred to as *girls* during this era), not only in terms of their fashion but also their attitude, was eventually dubbed the typical American girl.

Growth Charts: Growth charts refer to graphs kept by primary care providers on children as they age. Measurements are typically on height (or length in the case of infants) and weight. A child's measurements are compared to what is known to be typical of a child that age, and these measurements are presented in terms of percentiles.

Healthy Insurance Portability and Accountability Act (HIPAA): HIPAA was established in 1996 in the United States and regulates how private health information is stored and shared.

Heroin Chic: Heroin chic was a standard of beauty for women initially made popular by supermodel Kate Moss. This was an emaciated look that emphasized pale skin, dark circles under the eyes, and the angularity of bone structure.

Intuitive Eating: Intuitive eating refers to a philosophy and accompanying behaviors about eating that encourage people to rely on internal hunger and satiety cues with respect to when, how much, and what to eat.

Meta-Analysis: A meta-analysis is conducted in scientific research and refers to a study that examines the results of multiple studies that have already been conducted and that have looked at the same thing. The results of all of these studies are combined and analyzed statistically to see what the aggregate result is.

Metabolic Syndrome: Metabolic syndrome refers to a collection of health factors that can contribute to disease processes such as heart disease, diabetes, and stroke. There are five specific factors that put someone at risk for metabolic syndrome and having at least three of them results in a diagnosis of the syndrome. The five factors are having a large waistline, high triglycerides, low HDL cholesterol, high blood pressure, and high fasting blood sugar.

Muscular Ideal: The muscular ideal is the ideal body type for males which is described as a body that is lean clearly allowing muscle definition to show.

Obesity: Obesity generically refers to a body size that is larger than normal. Being identified as obese is done via measuring someone's BMI and then categorizing that BMI based on either CDC or WHO BMI categories. The obese category follows the overweight category and, according to the WHO, has three categories in and of itself: Class I Obesity, Class II Obesity, and Class III Obesity.

Overweight: Overweight refers to a body size that is larger than normal but not as larger as a body that is obese. Overweight is identified by measuring someone's BMI and then categorizing the BMI based on CDC or WHO BMI categories. The overweight category follows the normal weight category.

Reverse Causality: Also known as reverse causation, it refers to a cause-and-effect relationship between two factors that is not what would be expected. That is, one might assume a particular cause-and-effect relationship between two things but when they are studied it is revealed that the relationship between the two is the opposite of what was expected.

Thin Ideal: The thin ideal is the ideal currently emphasized for women's bodies. This ideal is depicted as being thin with a small waist and very little body fat.

TIMELINE

1800s	A fit male body is believed to reflect a high level of spirituality
1832	BMI is developed by Adolphe Quetelet but is called the Quetelet Index
1848	The first Woman's Rights Convention is held
1873	The Comstock Law makes it illegal to distribute anything indecent or salacious
Late 1800s	The male ideal is to be overweight, which is associated with wealth
Late 1800s/early 1900s	Looking like a Gibson Girl becomes the female ideal
Early 1900s	growth charts are first used to track normal or healthy growth in children
1900s	The popularity of magazines increases dramatically, among them the *Ladies' Home Journal*
1910s	Looking like a Fisher, Christy, or Brinkley Girl becomes the female ideal
August 19, 1920	The Nineteenth Amendment, granting women the right to vote, is ratified; Congress creates the Women's Bureau in the Department of Labor
1920s	Looking like a Flapper becomes the female ideal
	Fit and lean bodies as represented on the silver screen become the male ideal
1923	*Diet and Health, with Key to the Calories* by Lulu Hunt Peters becomes the first best-selling diet book, remaining in the position for four years

1929	The Flying Flapper, Elinor Smith, sets four world records in flying
1930s	Betty Boop first appears and is the first cartoon character to exhibit sexuality
	The *Hays Code* is applied to movies, and it regulates what is expected in terms of proper and moral behavior
1940s	"Rose the Riveter," a marketing image developed by the Office of War Information, becomes a female icon showing the strength and capabilities of women
	Willian Sheldon introduces the concepts of ectomorph, mesomorph, and endomorph to describe the bodies and personalities of men; the mesomorph body type is the ideal
Mid-1940s	Ancel Keys publishes his study entitled "Human Starvation and Its Consequences"
1946	The Centers for Disease Control and Prevention is founded
1948	The World Health Organization formally defines health
1950s	Marilyn Monroe, Betty Grable, and Lana Turner represent the female ideal
Mid-1950s	Audrey Hepburn becomes the female ideal
1959	The Barbie® doll is introduced
1960s	Bariatric surgery becomes a feasible method for losing weight, although surgery techniques pioneered in later decades will make the procedure safer and more effective
Mid-1960s	Twiggy (Leslie Hornsby) becomes the female ideal
1970s	Weight loss programs build franchises throughout the United States
1972	Ancel Keys formally renames the Quetelet Index of 1832 the body mass index (BMI) in his study entitled "Indices of Relative Weight and Obesity"
1977	The National Center for Health Sciences (NCHS) develops the NCHS Growth Charts
1978	The Centers for Disease Control and Prevention (CDC) applies a statistical procedure to the 1977 NCHS Growth Charts to normalize the expected growth curve for children, making the charts easier to use in practice
1980s	Cindy Crawford represents the female ideal
	Diet food becomes a new industry

1990s	Kate Moss becomes the female ideal and represents a standard eventually called "heroin chic"
1996	The United States introduces the Health Insurance Portability and Accountability Act, also known as HIPAA
1998	The Implicit Association Test (IAT) is published by Anthony Greenwald and Mahzarin Banaji
June 1998	The National Institutes of Health officially lowers the cutoff for overweight from a BMI of 27 to a BMI of 25
1999–2000	The CDC first publishes trends on obesity
2000	The CDC publishes a report calling for an update on growth charts; these charts are still used today and are the first version to include BMI as a measurement
2003	Arkansas becomes the first state to send home BMI report cards
2008	The book *Health at Every Size: The Surprising Truth about Your Weight* is published by Linda Bacon
February 9, 2010	Former First Lady Michelle Obama establishes the Let's Move! campaign designed to address childhood obesity
2012	The state of Georgia enacts a controversial ad campaign called *Stop Sugar Coating* in Georgia, which is designed to address childhood obesity
2013	The American Medical Association classifies obesity as a disease
2015	The Roadmap for Health Measurement and Accountability is established to identify best strategies for assessing health programs worldwide

SOURCES FOR FURTHER INFORMATION

ASSOCIATION FOR SIZE DIVERSITY AND HEALTH (ASDH)

http://www.sizediversityandhealth.org/

The Association for Size Diversity and Health was established in 2003 as an international professional organization. Its mission is to eradicate weight-related health policies and practices and to ensure that weight-related stigma is similarly abolished. They espouse the Health at Every Size® approach and encourage professional members to incorporate this approach in their practice.

CENTERS FOR DISEASE CONTROL AND PREVENTION (CDC)

https://www.cdc.gov

The website for the CDC is extensive and includes information on things such as Lyme disease, measles, stroke, heart disease, and obesity. Information on nearly any health issue that is of concern to citizens of the United States can be found here. The information incudes statistics on prevalence of the health issue, how to treat it, how to prevent it, and how to recognize it. Searching the term "obesity" in the website's search bar yields numerous links to internal information and resources.

COUNCIL ON SIZE AND WEIGHT DISCRIMINATION (CSWD)

www.cswd.org

This organization was established in 1991 and has the goals of changing public policies and societal attitudes regarding body weight. They offer information related to how the media portrays fat people, information for the press and for students, and information about kids and about being healthy. They also have a section of the website entitled "Bibliographies," which has links to books and articles on various topics related to weight, discrimination, and health.

EXERCISE IS MEDICINE® (EIM)

exerciseismedicine.org

The Exercise is Medicine® campaign was launched in 2007 by the American Medical Association (AMA) and the American College of Sports Medicine (ACSM). Although based in the United States, the two organizations intend it to be a global health initiative and currently have 43 centers around the world. The purpose of EIM is to encourage healthcare providers to include a measure of physical activity at every healthcare visit to determine, in part, if the patient is meeting the minimum requirements for physical activity. If not, the patient would be referred to other services, providers, and resources that can help them reach this minimum. The philosophy of EIM is that regular exercise has been consistently linked via scientific studies to being an effective form of treatment and prevention for myriad physical and mental health diseases. Links to the research are provided on the website.

HEALTH AT EVERY SIZE: THE SURPRISING TRUTH ABOUT YOUR WEIGHT

Author, Linda Bacon, PhD

This book, published in 2008, is an alternative and somewhat controversial approach to the traditional approach to weight loss. Dr. Bacon examines the research on myriad issues that affect one's overall weight and offers a method of moving away from dieting and toward a focus on healthy behaviors regardless of one's body weight, shape, or size.

LET'S MOVE!

https://letsmove.obamawhitehouse.archives.gov/

Let's Move! was the initiative of former first lady, Michelle Obama, which was developed for the explicit purpose of addressing the "epidemic of childhood obesity," and launched on February 9, 2010. The website includes information about childhood obesity, eating healthy, ways to be physically active, and information for those who interact with children and who want to help address childhood obesity. The Let's Move! website comprised of information many readers may find useful, but it is no longer active. The information is no longer updated and therefore should not be considered current and may need to be verified elsewhere for its veracity. The top of the website has a disclaimer that says "This is historical material 'frozen in time.' The website is no longer updated and links to external websites and some internal pages may not work."

NATIONAL ASSOCIATION TO ADVANCE FAT ACCEPTANCE (NAAFA)

https://www.naafaonline.com/dev2/
NAAFA is a civil rights organization that was established in 1969. Its purpose is to work through advocacy and education to end size discrimination. They offer support to and tools for fat people so they can advocate for and empower themselves. The organization currently offers free webinars and links to information about HAES®, bullying and discrimination.

OBESITY ACTION COALITION (OAC)

www.obesityaction.org
The Obesity Action Coalition is an organization with over 50,000 members. This organization is dedicated to helping those affected by obesity which they refer to as a disease. Their goals involve education and awareness around obesity as a disease and helping people get access to obesity treatment and prevention efforts while also working to eliminate weight bias and discrimination. The website includes pages offering information on obesity in general, obesity in children, information on weight bias, and information on resources both locally and nationally. They also provide links to printable brochures and guides that are free to download in pdf format and can be printed.

PROJECT IMPLICIT

https://implicit.harvard.edu/implicit/takeatest.html
Project Implicit is a website where you can take any number of tests on implicit attitudes or biases (i.e., biases that we may not be consciously aware of). This project was established in 1998 by researchers from Harvard University, the University of Washington, and the University of Virginia. In addition to Implicit Association Tests on things such as religion, race, age, disability, gender, and other demographics, Project Implicit also provides consultation, workshops, and other services designed to address biases, inclusion, and diversity.

RUDD CENTER FOR FOOD POLICY AND OBESITY

http://www.uconnruddcenter.org/
The Rudd Center for Food Policy and Obesity is connected with the University of Connecticut. Their aim is to address childhood obesity via awareness and education around eating behaviors and by addressing weight bias. Their efforts include helping to ensure public policies are informed by science. They provide information for and work with families and communities, schools, agencies writing public policy, and food marketing.

U.S. NATIONAL PHYSICAL ACTIVITY GUIDELINES (PAG)

https://health.gov/paguidelines/guidelines/
The U.S. National Physical Activity Guidelines are provided by the governmental Office of Disease Prevention and Health Promotion. The guidelines themselves can be read online or can be downloaded, printed, and shared for free in pdf format. The current guidelines on this site were published in 2008.

WORLD HEALTH ORGANIZATION (WHO)

http://www.who.int/en/
The World Health Organization is devoted to addressing health-related issues that affect people around the world. They are located in over 150 countries and work with local governments and other agencies invested in ensuring a healthy population. They work to try to prevent the spread of, provide treatment for, and prevent infectious diseases (e.g., flu, HIV) and noncommunicable diseases (e.g., cancer, heart disease). Searching the term "obesity" into their search bar yields over 13,000 results that include information on obesity itself (e.g., statistics), obesity's connection to other health-related concerns, information related to economics and obesity, and so on.

BIBLIOGRAPHY

Afzal, Shoaib, Anne Tybaerg-Hansen, Grom B. Jensen, and Børge G. Nordestgaard. "Change in Body Mass Index Associated with Lowest Mortality in Denmark, 1976–2013." *Journal of the American Medical Association* 315 (2016): 1989–96.

Ahima, Rexford S., and Mitchell A. Lazar. "The Health Risk of Obesity—Better Metrics Imperative." *Science* 341 (2013): 856–58.

American Liver Foundation. "NAFLD: Non-Alcoholic Fatty Liver Disease." *American Liver Foundation*, accessed May 5, 2017, http://www.liverfoundation.org/abouttheliver/info/nafld/.

Armstrong, Ruth. "Obesity, Law and Personal Responsibility." *The Medical Journal of Australia* 186 (2007): 20.

Arthritis Foundation. "Osteoarthritis." *Arthritis Foundation*, accessed May 5, 2017, http://www.arthritis.org/about-arthritis/types/osteoarthritis/.

Bacon, Linda. *Health at Every Size: The Surprising Truth about Your Weight*. Dallas: Benbella Books, 2008.

Bacon, Linda, and Lucy Aphramor. "Weight Science: Evaluating the Evidence for a Paradigm Shift." *Nutrition Journal* 10 (2011): 1–13.

Baird, I. M. "Obesity and Insurance Risk: The Insurance Industry's Viewpoint." *Pharmacoeconomics*, 5 (1994): 62–65.

Ballman, Donna. "Is Weight Discrimination at Work Illegal?" *Aol Jobs*, accessed February 24, 2016, http://jobs.aol.com/articles/2012/11/06/is-weight-discrimination-illegal/.

Barker, D. J. P. "Fetal Origins of Coronary Heart Disease." *British Medical Journal* 311 (1995): 171–74.

Bastien, Marjorie, Paul Poirier, Isabelle Lemieux, and Jean-Pierre Després. "Overview of Epidemiology and Contribution of Obesity to Cardiovascular Disease." *Progress in Cardiovascular Diseases* 56 (2014): 369–81.

Berman, Margit I., Stephanie N. Morton, and Mark T. Hegel. "Health at Every Size and Acceptance and Commitment Therapy for Obese, Depressed Women: Treatment Development and Clinical Application." *Clinical Social Work Journal* 44 (2016): 265–78.

Blackburn, Henry, and David Jacobs Jr. "Commentary: Origins and Evolution of Body Mass Index (BMI): Continuing Saga." *International Journal of Epidemiology* 43 (2014): 665–69.

Bombak, Andrea. "Obesity, Health at Every Size, and Public Health Policy." *American Journal of Public Health,* 104 (2014): e60–67.

Bonfiglioli, Catriona, M. F., Ben J. Smith, Lesley A. King, Simon F. Chapman, and Simon J. Holding. "Choice and Voice: Obesity Debates in Television News." *Medical Journal of Australian* 187 (2007): 442–45.

Boone, Liesbet, Bart Soenens, and Carolline Braet. "Perfectionism, Body Dissatisfaction, and Bulimic Symptoms: The Intervening Role of Perceived Pressure to Be Thin and Thin Ideal Internalization." *Journal of Social and Clinical Psychology* 30 (2011): 1043–68.

Brickman, P., D. Coates, and R. Janoff-Bulman. "Lottery Winners and Accident Victims: Is Happiness Relative?" *Journal of Personality and Social Psychology* 36 (1978): 287–302.

Brooks, Benjamin. "Personal Responsibility or Shared Responsibility: What Is the Appropriate Role in the Law in Obesity Prevention?" *Journal of Law and Medicine* 23 (2015): 106-20.

Burgard, Deborah. "What's Weight Got to Do with It? Weight Neutrality in the Health at Every Size Paradigm and Its Implications for Clinical Practice." In *Treatment of Eating Disorders: Bridging the Research-Practice Gap,* edited by Margo Maine, Beth Hartman McGilley and Douglas W. Bunnell, 17–35. Boston: Elsevier, 2010.

Callahan, Daniel. "Obesity: Chasing an Elusive Epidemic." *Hastings Center Report.* January-February 2013: 34–40.

Campaign to End Obesity. "Obesity Facts & Resources." *obesitycampaign.org,* accessed March 10, 2017. http://www.obesitycampaign.org/obesity_facts.asp.

Cara, Ed. "Heath at Every Size Movement: What Proponents Say vs. What Science Says." *Medicaldaily.com.* April 22, 2016. http://www.medicaldaily.com/health-every-size-obesity-weight-loss-science-383008.

Centers for Disease Control and Prevention. "Adult Obesity Prevalence Maps." *cdc.gov.* April 10, 2017. https://www.cdc.gov/obesity/data/prevalence-maps.html

Centers for Disease Control and Prevention. "Prevalence of Childhood Obesity in the United States, 2011–2014." *cdc.gov.* April 10, 2017. https://www.cdc.gov/obesity/data/childhood.html

Chastain, Ragen. "Are Fat People Really Oppressed?" *DancesWithFat.wordpress.com.* May 9, 2014. https://danceswithfat.wordpress.com/2014/05/09/are-fat-people-really-oppressed-2/.

Chenoweth, D. H., R. C. Rager, and R. G. Haynes. "Relationship between Body Mass Index and Workers' Compensation Claims and Costs: Results from the

North Carolina's League of Municipalities Database." *Journal of Occupational and Environmental Medicine,* 57 (2015): 931–37.

Choban, Patricia S., Steve Poplawski, Benita Jackson, and Peter Bistolarides. "Bariatric Surgery for Morbid Obesity: Why, Who, When, How, Where, and Then What?" *Cleveland Clinic Journal of Medicine* 69 (2002): 897–903.

CNN. "Who's Fat? New Definition Adopted." *CNN.com.* June 17, 1998. www.cnn.com/HEALTH/9806/17/weight.guidelines/.

Common Road Map Steering Committee. *The Roadmap for Health Measurement and Accountability.* Washington, D.C.: MA4Health, 2015.

Cossrow, Nicole, and Bonita Falkner. "Race/Ethnic Issues in Obesity and Obesity-Related Comorbidities." *The Journal of Clinical Endocrinology & Metabolism* 89 (2004): 2590–94.

Curioni, C. C., and P. M. Lourenço. "Long-Term Weight Loss after Diet and Exercise: A Systematic Review." *International Journal of Obesity* 29 (2005): 1168–74.

Danielsdottir, Sigrun, Deb Burgard, and Wendy Oliver-Pyatt. "Guidelines for Childhood Obesity Prevention Programs." *Academy for Eating Disorders.* February 26, 2009, http://www.aedweb.org/index.php/23-get-involved/position-statements/90-aed-statement-on-body-shaming-and-weight-prejudice-in-public-endeavors-to-reduce-obesity-4.

Dee, Anne, Karen Kearns, Ciaran O'Neill, Linda Sharp, Anthony Staines, Victoria O'Dwyer, Sarah Fitzgerald, and Ivan J. Perry. "The Direct and Indirect Costs of Both Overweight and Obesity: A Systematic Review." *BioMed Central Research Notes* 7 (2014): 242.

Dombrowski, S. U., K. Knittle, A. Avelnell, V. Araújo-Soares, and F. F. Sniehotta. "Long Term Maintenance of Weight Loss with Non-Surgical Interventions in Obese Adults: Systematic Review and Meta-Analyses of Randomised Controlled Trials." *British Medical Journal* 348 (2014): g2646.

Douketis, J. D., C. Macie, L. Thabane, and D. F. Williamson. "Systematic Review of Long-Term Weight Loss Studies in Obese Adults Clinical Significance and Applicability to Clinical Practice." *International Journal of Obesity* 29 (2005): 1153–67.

Duchovny, Noelia, and Colin Baker. "How Does Obesity in Adults Affect Spending on Health Care?" *Economic and Budget Issue Brief,* September 8, 2010, accessed April 17, 2017, https://www.cbo.gov/sites/default/files/cbofiles/ftpdocs/118xx/doc11810/09-08-obesity_brief.pdf.

Ebbeling, Cara, B., Dorota B. Pawlak, and David S. Ludwig. "Childhood Obesity: Public-Health Crisis, Common Sense Cure." *The Lancet* 360 (2002): 473–82.

Economist, The. "Pots of Promise: The Beauty Promise." *The Economist.* May 22, 2003. http://www.economist.com/node/1795852

Eknoyan, Garabed. "Adolphe Quetelet (1796–1874)—The Average Man and Indices of Obesity." *Nephrol Dial Transplant* 23 (2008): 47–51.

Fabbrini, Elisa, Shelby Sullivan, and Samuel Klein. "Obesity and Nonalcoholic Fatty Liver Disease: Biochemical, Metabolic and Clinical Implications." *Hepatology* 51 (2010): 679-89.

Flegal, Katherine M., Barry I. Graubard, David F. Williamson, and Mitchell H. Gail. "Excess Deaths Associated with Underweight, Overweight, and Obesity." *Journal of the American Medical Association* 293 (2005): 1861–67.

Flegal, Katherine M., Brian K. Kit, Heather Orpana, and Barry I. Graubard. "Association of All-Cause Mortality with Overweight and Obesity Using Standard Body Mass Index Categories: A Systematic Review and Meta-Analysis." *Journal of the American Medical Association* 309 (2013): 71–82.

Frellick, Marcia. "AMA Declares Obesity a Disease." *Medscape*. June 19, 20013. http://www.medscape.com/viewarticle/806566.

Gaesser, Glenn A. *Big Fat Lies: The Truth About Your Weight and Your Health*. Carlsbad: Gürze Books, 2002.

Gee, Kevin A. "School-Based Body Mass Index Screening and Parental Notification in Late Adolescence: Evidence from Arkansas's Act 1220." *Journal of Adolescent Health* 57 (2015): 270–76.

Geier, Andrew B., Gary D. Foster, Leslie G. Womble, Jackie McLaughlin, Kelley E. Borradaile, Joan Nachamani, Sandy Sherman, Shiriki Kumanyika, and Justine Shults. "The Relationship between Relative Weight and School Attendance among Elementary Schoolchildren." *Obesity* 15 (2007): 2157–61.

Gilbert, Daniel T., Elizabeth C. Pinel, Timothy D. Wilson, Stephen J. Blumberg, and Thalia P. Wheatley. "Immune Neglect: A Source of Durability Bias in Affective Forecasting." *Journal of Personality and Social Psychology* 75 (1998): 617–38.

Gosse, A. Hope. "Obesity from the Point of View of the Insurance Medical Officer." *The Medical Press* 228 (1952): 488–91.

Gostin, Lawrence O. "Law as a Tool to Facilitate Healthier Lifestyles and Prevent Obesity." *Journal of the American Medical Association* 297 (2007): 87–90.

Gourley, Catherine. *Flappers and the New American Woman: Perceptions of Women from 1918 through the 1920s*. Minneapolis: Twenty-First Century Books, 2008.

Gourley, Catherine. *Gibson Girls and Suffragists: Perceptions of Women from 1900 to 1918*. Minneapolis: Twenty-First Century Books, 2008.

Gourley, Catherine. *Gidgets and Women Warriors: Perceptions of Women in the 1950s and 1960s*. Minneapolis: Twenty-First Century Books, 2008.

Gourley, Catherine. *Ms. and the Material Girls: Perceptions of Women from the 1970s through the 1990s*. Minneapolis: Twenty-First Century Books, 2008.

Gourley, Catherine. *Rosie and Mrs. America: Perceptions of Women in the 1930s and 1940s*. Minneapolis: Twenty-First Century Books, 2008.

Gracia-Marco, Luis, Luis A. Moreno, and German Vicente-Rodriguez. "Impact of Social Marketing in the Prevention of Childhood Obesity." *Advances in Nutrition* 3 (2012): 611S-615S.

GRADE Workgroup. "What Is GRADE?" *gradeworkinggroup.org*, accessed March 1, 2017. www.gradeworkinggroup.org.

Greenberg, James A. "Correcting Biases in Estimates of Mortality Attributable to Obesity." *Obesity* 14 (2006): 2071–79.

Greenfield, Beth. "Shocking Anti-Obesity PSA Sparks Debate." *Yahoo.com.* October 16, 2014. https://www.yahoo.com/parenting/shocking-anti-obesity-psa-sparks-debate- 94551060722.html.

Griffiths, Scott, Stuart B. Murray, and Stephen Touyz. "Disordered Eating and the Muscular Ideal." *Journal of Eating Disorders* 1 (2013): 15.

Grinberg, Emanuella. "Georgia's Child Obesity Ads Aim to Create Movement out of Controversy." *CNN.com.* February 7, 2012. http://www.cnn.com/2012/02/07/health/atlanta-child-obesity-ads/.

Guyatt, Gordon H., Andrew D. Oxman, Gunn E. Vist, Regina Kunz, Yngve Falck-Ytter, Pablo Alonso-Coello, and Holder J. Schünemann. "GRADE: An Emerging Consensus on Rating Quality of Evidence and Strength of Recommendations." *British Medical Journal* 336 (2008): 924–26.

Hamer, Mark, and Emmanuel Stamatakis. "Metabolically Healthy Obesity and Risk of All-Cause and Cardiovascular Disease Mortality." *Journal of Clinical Endocrinology & Metabolism* 97 (2012): 2482–88.

Hammermesh, Daniel S., and Jason Abrevaya. "Beauty Is the Promise of Happiness?" *Institute for the Study of Labor*, March 2011 (IZA DP No. 5600).

Hatzenbuehler, Mark L., Katherine M. Keyes, and Deborah S. Hasin. "Associations between Perceived Weight Discrimination and the Prevalence of Psychiatric Disorders in the General Population." *Obesity* 17 (2009): 2033–39.

Humphrey, Lauren, Dawn Clifford, and Michelle Neyman Morris. "*Health at Every Size* College Course Reduces Dieting Behaviors and Improves Intuitive Eating, Body Esteem, and Anti-Fat Attitudes." *Journal of Nutrition Education and Behavior,* 47 (2015): 354–60.

Kaczmarek, Lukasz D., Jolanta Enko, Malgorzata Awdziejczyk, Natalia Hoffman, Natalia Bialobrzeska, Przemyslaw Mielniczuk, and Stephan U. Dombrowski. "Would You Be Happier if You Looked Better? A Focusing Illusion." *Journal of Happiness Studies* 17 (2016): 357–65.

Kelly, Inas Rashad, and Sara Markowitz. "Incentives in Obesity and Health Insurance." *Inquiry* 46 (2009): 418–32.

Kersh, Rogan. "The Politics of Obesity: A Current Assessment and Look Ahead." *The Milbank Quarterly* 87 (2009): 295–316.

Keys, Ancel. "Human Starvation and Its Consequences." *American Dietetic Association* 22 (1946): 582–87.

Kopelman, Peter. G. "Obesity as a Medical Problem." *Nature* 404 (2000): 635–43.

Krashnewski, Jennifer L., J. Boan, J. Esposito, N. E. Sherwook, E. B. Lehman, D. K. Kephart, and C. N. Sciamanna. "Long-Term Weight Loss Maintenance in the United States." *International Journal of Obesity* 34 (2010): 1644–54.

Landhuis, Esther. "Healthiest Weight Just Might Be 'Overweight.' " *ScienceNews.org.* May 11, 2016. https://www.sciencenews.org/article/healthy-weight-bmi-overweight.

Lang, Astrid, and Erika Sivarajan Froelicher. "Management of Overweight and Obesity in Adults: Behavioral Intervention for Long-Term Weight Loss and Maintenance." *European Journal of Cardiovascular Nursing* 5 (2006): 102–14.

Langlois, Judith H., Lisa Kalakanis, Adam J. Rubenstein, Andrea Larson, Monica
    Hallam, and Monica Smoot. "Maxims or Myths of Beauty? A Meta-Analytic
    and Theoretical Review." *Psychological Bulletin* 126 (2000): 390–423.
Luft, Vivian C., Maria I. Schmidt, James S. Pankow, David Couper, Christie M.
    Ballantyne, J. Hunter Young, and Bruce B. Duncan. "Chronic Inflammation
    Role in the Obesity-Diabetes Association: A Case-Cohort Study." *Diabetol-
    ogy & Metabolic Syndrome* 5 (2013): 31.
Madsen, Kristine A. "School-Based BMI Screening and Parent Notification:
    A Statewide Natural Experiment." *Archives of Pediatrics and Adolescent
    Medicine* 165 (2011): 987–92.
Mann, Traci, A. Janet Tomiyama, Erika Westling, Ann-Marie Lew, Barbra
    Samuels, and Jason Chatman. "Medicare's Search for Effective Obesity
    Treatments: Diets Are Not the Answer." *American Psychologist* 63 (2007):
    220–33.
Mariner, Wendy K. "Social Solidarity and Personal Responsibility in Health
    Reform." *Connecticut Insurance Law Journal* 14 (2008): 199–228.
Mello, Michelle M., David M. Studdert, and Troyen A. Brennan. "Obesity—The
    New Frontier of Public Health Law." *The New England Journal of Medicine*
    354 (2006): 2601–10.
Mensah, George A., Richard A. Goodman, Stephanie Zaza, Anthony D. Moulton,
    Paula L. Kocher, William H. Dietz, Terry F. Pechacek, and James S. Marks.
    "Law as a Tool for Preventing Chronic Diseases: Expanding the Spectrum
    of Effective Public Health Strategies." *Preventing Chronic Disease: Public
    Health Research, Practice and Policy* 1 (1) (2004): 1–8.
National Association to Advance Fat Acceptance. "Facts on Size Discrimina-
    tion." *naafaonline.com,* accessed February 24, 2016 http://www.naafaonline
    .com/dev2/assets/documents/naafa_FactSheet_v17_screen.pdf.
National Cancer Institute. "Obesity and Cancer." *National Institute of Health:
    National Cancer Institute,* accessed May 5, 2017. https://www.cancer.gov/
    about-cancer/causes-prevention/risk/obesity/obesity-fact-sheet.
National Heart, Lung, and Blood Institute. "What Is Metabolic Syndrome?"
    National Institute of Health: National Heart, Lung and Blood Institute.
    June 22, 2016. https://www.nhlbi.nih.gov/health/health-topics/topics/ms.
NCHS. "Prevalence of Obesity among Adults and Youth: United States, 2011–
    2014." *NCHS Data Brief No. 219.* November 2015, accessed February 27,
    2016, http://www.cdc.gov/nchs/data/databriefs/db219.htm.
Nestle, Marion. "The Ironic Politics of Obesity." *Science* 299 (2003): 781.
Neumark-Sztainer, Dianne, Melanie Wall, Jess Haines, Mary Story, and Marla E.
    Eisenberg. "Why Does Dieting Predict Weight Gain in Adolescents? Find-
    ings from Project EAT-II: A 5-Year Longitudinal Study." *Journal of the
    American Dietetic Association* 107 (2007): 448–55.
NPR. "Controversy Swirls Around Harsh Anti-Obesity Ads." *NPR.org.* January 9,
    2012. http://www.npr.org/2012/01/09/144799538/controversy-swirls-around-
    harsh-anti-obesity-ads.

O'Brien, Kerry S., Janet D. Latner, Lenny R. Vartanian, Claudia Giles, Konstadina Griva, and Adrian Carter. "The Relationship between Weight Stigma and Eating Behaviors Is Explained by Weight Bias Internalization and Psychological Distress." *Appetite* 102 (2016): 70–76.

Ogden, Cynthia L., Molly M. Lamb, Margaret D. Carroll, and Katherine M. Flegal. "Obesity and Socioeconomic Status in Adults: United States 2005–2008." *NCHS Data Brief, No. 50*. Hyattsville, MD: National Center for Health Statistics, 2010.

Ogden, Cynthia L., Molly M. Lamb, Margaret D. Carroll, and Katherine M. Flegal. "Obesity and Socioeconomic Status in Children: United States 1988–1994 and 2005–2008." *NCHS Data Brief, No. 51*. Hyattsville, MD: National Center for Health Statistics, 2010.

Ogden, Cynthia L., Margaret D. Carroll, Cheryl D. Fryer, and Katherine M. Flegal. "Prevalence of Obesity among Adults and Youth in the United States, 2011–2014." *NCHS Data Brief, No. 219*. Hyattsville, MD: National Center for Health Statistics, 2015.

Ogden, Cynthia L., Margaret D. Carroll, Brian K. Kit, and Katherine M. Flegal. "Prevalence of Childhood and Adult Obesity in the United States, 2011–2012." *Journal of the American Medical Association* 311 (2014): 806–14.

Padula, W. V., R. R. Allen, and K. V. Nair. "Determining the Cost of Obesity and Its Common Comorbidities from a Commercial Claims Database." *Clinical Obesity* 4 (2013): 53–58.

Pan, L., B. Sherry, S Park, and H. M. Blanck. "The Association of Obesity and School Absenteeism Attributed to Illness or Injury Among Adolescents in the United States, 2009." *The Journal of Adolescent Health* 52 (2013): 64–69.

Penney, Tarra L., and Sara F. L. Kirk. "The Health at Every Size Paradigm and Obesity: Missing Empirical Evidence May Help Push the Reframing Obesity Debate Forward." *American Journal of Public Health,* 105 (2015): e38–42.

Pennman, Alan D., and William D. Johnson. "The Changing Shape of the Body Mass Index Distribution Curve in the Population: Implications for Public Health Policy to Reduce the Prevalence of Adult Obesity." *Preventing Chronic Disease: Public Health Research, Practice, and Policy* 3 (2006): 1–4.

Preamble to the Constitution of the World Health Organization as Adopted by the International Health Conference, New York, June 19–22, 1946; signed on July 22, 1946, by the representatives of 61 States (Official Records of the World Health Organization, no. 2, p. 100) and entered into force on April 7, 1948.

Prospective Studies Collaboration. "Body-Mass Index and Cause-Specific Mortality in 900,000 Adults: Collaborative Analyses of 57 Prospective Studies." *The Lancet* 37 (2009): 1083–96.

Provencher, Véronique, Catherine Bégin, Angelo Tremblay, Lyne Mongeau, Sonia Boivin, and Simone Lemieux. "Short-Term Effects of a 'Health-At-Every-Size Approach on Eating Behaviors and Appetite Ratings." *Obesity* 15 (2007): 957–66.

Puhl, Rebecca M., and Chelsea A. Heuer. "Obesity Stigma: Important Consid-
    erations for Public Health." *American Journal of Public Health* 100 (2010):
    1019–28.
Puhl, Rebecca M., and Chelsea A. Heuer. "The Stigma of Obesity: A Review and
    Update." *Obesity* 17 (2009): 941–64.
Puhl, Rebecca M., and Janet D. Latner. "Sigma, Obesity, and the Health of the
    Nation's Children." *Psychological Bulletin* 133 (2007): 557–90.
Robertson, Noelle, and Reena Vohora. "Fitness vs. Fatness: Implicit Bias towards
    Obesity among Fitness Professionals and Regular Exercisers." *Psychology of
    Sport and Exercise* 9 (2008): 547–57.
Rudd Center for Food Policy and Obesity. *Rudd Report: Weight Bias: A Social Jus-
    tice Issue.* New Haven, CT: Rudd Center for Food Policy and Obesity, 2009.
Sainsbury, Amanda, and Phillipa Hay. "Call for an Urgent Rethink of the 'Health
    at Every Size' Concept." *Journal of Eating Disorders,* 2 (2014): 1–4.
Schkade, David A., and Daniel Kahneman. "Does Living in California Make
    People Happy?: A Focusing Illusion in Judgments of Life Satisfaction." *Psy-
    chological Science* 9 (1998): 340–45.
Schmidt, Harald. "Obesity and Blame: Elusive Goals for Personal Responsibil-
    ity." *Hastings Center Report.* May–June 2013: 8–9.
Shore, Stuart M., Michael L. Sachs, Jeffrey R. Lidicker, Stephanie N. Brett,
    Adam R. Wright, and Joseph R. Libonati. "Decreased Scholastic Achieve-
    ment in Overweight Middle School Students." *Obesity* 16 (2008): 1535–38.
Simmons-Duffin, Selena. "New Anti-Obesity Ads Blaming Overweight Par-
    ents Sparks Criticism." *NPR.org.* September 27, 2012 http://www.npr.org/
    sections/thesalt/2012/09/27/161831449/new-anti-obesity-ads-blaming-
    overweight-parents-spark-criticism.
Small, Jennie, and Candice Harris. "Obesity and Tourism: Rights and Responsi-
    bilities." *Annals of Tourism Research* 39 (2012): 686–707.
State of Obesity, The. "The Healthcare Costs of Obesity." *Stateofobesity.org,*
    accessed March 10, 2017 http://stateofobesity.org/healthcare-costs-obesity/.
Statista.com. "Revenue of the Cosmetic/Beauty Industry in the United States
    from 2002–2016 (in Billion U.S. Dollars)." *Statista.com,* accessed January
    5, 2017 https://www.statista.com/statistics/243742/revenue-of-the-cosmetic-
    industry-in-the-us/.
Statista.com. "Size of Total Weight Loss Market in the U.S. from 2013–2015 (in
    Billion U.S. Dollars)." *Statista.com,* accessed January 6, 2017 https://www
    .statista.com/statistics/625673/total-weight-loss-market-size-in-us/.
Statista.com. "Total Expenditure on Cosmetic Procedures in the United States in
    2015, by Type (in Billion U.S. Dollars)." *Statista.com,* accessed January 6,
    2017 https://www.statista.com/statistics/281346/total-expenditure-on-
    cosmetic-procedures-in-the-united-states-by-type/.
Stice, Eric, and Katherine Presnell. *The Body Project: Promoting Body Accep-
    tance and Preventing Eating Disorders.* New York: Oxford University Press,
    2007.

Stokes, Rachel, and Christina Frederick-Recascino. "Women's Perceived Body Image: Relations with Personal Happiness." *Journal of Women and Aging* 15 (2003): 17–29.

Swami, Viren, Ulrich S. Tran, Stefan Stieger, and Martin Voracek. "Associations between Women's Body Image and Happiness: Results of the YouBeauty.com Body Image Survey (YBIS)." *Journal of Happiness Studies* 16 (2015): 705–18.

Thacker, Stephen B., Donna F. Stroup, Vilma Carande-Kulis, James S. Marks, Kakoli Roy, and Julie L. Gerberding. "Measuring the Public's Health." *Public Health Reports* 121 (2006): 14–22.

Thompson, Kevin J., and Eric Stice. "Thin-Ideal Internalization: Mounting Evidence for a New Risk Factor for Body-Image Disturbance and Eating Pathology." *Current Directions in Psychological Science* 10 (2001): 181–83.

Unger, Roger H., and Phillipp E. Scherer. "Gluttony, Sloth and the Metabolic Syndrome: A Roadmap to Lipotoxicity." *Trends in Endocrinology & Metabolism* 21 (2010): 345–52.

USA Today. "College Requires Heavy Students to Take Fitness Class to Graduate." *usatoday.com.* November 23, 2009. http://usatoday30.usatoday.com/news/health/weightloss/2009-11-23-college-obesity_N.htm.

U.S. Census Bureau. "How the Census Bureau Measures Poverty." *census.gov,* accessed February 28, 2016 https://www.census.gov/hhes/www/poverty/about/overview/measure.html.

U.S. Department of Health and Human Services. "Bariatric Surgery for Severe Obesity." *Weight-Control Information Network Fact Sheet (June 2011),* accessed February 29, 2016 http://www.niddk.nih.gov/health-information/health-topics/weight-control/bariatric-surgery-severe-obesity/Documents/Bariatric_Surgery_508.pdf.

U.S. Department of Health and Human Services. "Prescription Medications for the Treatment of Obesity." *Weight-Control Information Network Fact Sheet (April 2013),* accessed February 29, 2016 http://www.sumnerdietrx.com/files/2013/03/Prescription_Medications.pdf.

U.S. Equal Employment Opportunity Commission. "Facts about Discrimination in Federal Government Employment Based on Marital Status, Political Affiliation, Status as a Parent, Sexual Orientation, and Gender Identity." *U.S. Equal Employment Opportunity Commission,* accessed February 24, 2016 http://www.eeoc.gov/federal/otherprotections.cfm.

Vigen, Tyler. "Spurious Correlations." *tylervigen.com,* accessed February 18, 2016. http://tylervigen.com/spurious-correlations.

Vogel, Lauren. "The Skinny on BMI Report Cards." *Canadian Medical Association Journal* 183 (2011): E787–88.

Waller, Bruce N. "Responsibility and Health." *Cambridge Quarterly of Healthcare Ethics,* 14 2005): 177–88.

Wang, S. S., K. D. Brownell, and T. A. Wadden. "The Influence of the Stigma of Obesity on Overweight Individuals." *International Journal of Obesity* 28 (2004): 1333–37.

Williams, Ellen P., Marie Mesidor, Karen Winters, Patricia M. Dubbert, and Sharon B. Wyatt. "Overweight and Obesity: Prevalence, Consequences, and Causes of a Growing Public Health Problem." *Current Obesity Reports* 4 (2015): 363–70.

Wing, R. R., and James O. Hill. "Successful Weight Loss Maintenance." *Annual Review of Nutrition* 21 (2001): 323–41.

Wing, R. R., and Suzanne Phelan. "Long-Term Weight Loss Maintenance." *American Journal of Clinical Nutrition* 82 (suppl) (2005): 222S–25S.

INDEX

Academy for Eating Disorders
      (AED), 52–53
Adjustable gastric band (AGB),
      62–63
Adolescents, 16, 28, 42–44, 47–48,
      52, 62, 123, 147–48, 175
Adults, 22, 29, 38, 42–45, 47–48, 53,
      59–62, 80–81, 83, 100, 113,
      120, 122, 128, 134, 138, 147,
      154, 169, 175
Affective forecasting, 105
All-cause mortality, 128–31. *See also*
      Mortality rate
Alli, 60
American Academy of Pediatrics,
      27, 52
American Liver Foundation
      (ALF), 114
American Medical Association
      (AMA), 119, 145, 185, 188;
      *Journal of American Medical
      Association*, 129
Anorexia nervosa, 10, 19–20,
      25–26, 70
Anti-fat bias: and access to services,
      73–79; and airlines, 74–76; and
      cultural and political attitudes,
      79–85; and education, 79; and
      effects on treatment, 70–72;
      and effects on well-being,
      70–72; and fitness and
      exercise facilities, 76–77;
      and internalization, 83–85;
      and medical care, 66–70; and
      medical services, 77–78; and
      physical health, 82–83; and
      psychological effects, 80–82;
      and other public services,
      78–79; what is, 65–66. *See also*
      Size discrimination; Weight bias
Anxiety, 70, 80–81, 136
Arden, Elizabeth, 7

Bacon, Linda, 88–94, 185, 188. *See
      also* Health at Every Size®
      (HAES®)
Barbie® doll, 10–11, 184
Bariatric surgery, 33–34, 57, 59,
      61–64, 113, 171, 179, 184. *See
      also* Weight loss surgery; *and
      specific types of weight loss
      surgeries*
Basal metabolic rate, 36. *See also*
      Metabolism

Beauty industry, 106
Behavior management, 57, 59
Bell curve, 38. *See also* Normal
     curve; Normal distribution
Belly fat, 117
Belviq, 60
Bezphetamine, 60. *See
     also* Diethylpropion;
     Phendimetrazine; Phentermine
Bigorexia, 19. *See also* Muscle
     dysmorphia
Biliopancreatic diversion with a
     duodenal switch (BPD-DS),
     62–63
Binge eating disorder (BED), 19,
     70, 82
Blood pressure, 34, 59, 71, 83,
     93–94, 112, 117, 127, 151, 157,
     172, 180
Blood sugar, 59, 71, 110–11, 117,
     157, 172, 180. *See also* Glucose
BMI, 21, 41, 65, 109, 169, 174,
     176–77, 180–81, 183–85;
     and ad campaigns, 49–51;
     and age, 42–43; and behavior
     management, 57–58; and
     cardiovascular disease, 112;
     and CDC and public health
     policy, 53–54; and control
     of, 35–37; and costs, 39–33,
     134–35; and diabetes, 110–11;
     and education level, 48–49;
     and growth charts and medical
     records, 27–29; and Health
     at Every Size®, 89, 91, 151,
     155–57; and health insurance,
     29–35; and income level,
     46–48; and life expectancy,
     128–31; and long-term
     weight loss, 123–24; and
     medication therapy, 59–61; and
     nonalcoholic fatty liver disease,
     114; and normal (bell) curve,
     38–40; and one-size-fits-all
approach, dangers of, 72–73;
     and origin and definition of,
     24–27, 179; and political
     attitudes, 54–56; and
     psychological effects of, 81;
     and questioning the research,
     116–18; and race/ethnicity,
     44–46; and report cards, 151,
     156, 165–67, 179; and school
     policies, 51–53; and sex,
     43–44; and size discrimination,
     56–57; and weight loss surgery,
     61–64, 171. *See also* Obesity;
     Overweight
BMI Report Cards, 41, 51, 156,
     179, 185
Body fat, 17–18, 71, 95, 110–11, 113,
     116–17, 181
Body mass index. *See* BMI
*Body Project: Promoting
     Body Acceptance and
     Preventing Eating
     Disorders, The*, 100
Body shape and size, 11, 18–20, 52,
     56–57, 65, 69, 96, 99, 138, 144,
     152, 156, 160. *See also* Body
     weight
Body type, 3, 12, 14–15, 17, 99,
     158–59, 180, 184. *See also*
     Muscular ideal; Thin ideal
Body weight, 19, 59, 89, 96, 119–20,
     123, 139, 142, 144, 156, 158,
     160, 187–88. *See also* Body
     shape and size
Boop, Betty, 8, 184
Brain, 36–37, 60, 62, 114
Brinkley, Nell, 5. *See also*
     Brinkley Girls
Brinkley Girls, 5, 183
Bulimia nervosa, 19–20, 70, 82

Calories, 7, 12, 19, 34–37, 53,
     57, 63, 87, 93, 119–20,
     168, 170, 173, 176

Carbon dioxide, 113–14. *See also* Sleep apnea
Cardiovascular disease, 111–12, 117, 127, 129, 131, 135, 173–74
Cause and effect, 32–33, 104, 116, 126, 130, 181. *See also* Correlation
Cause-specific mortality, 128. *See also* All-cause mortality; Mortality rate
Census Bureau, United States, 47
Centers for Disease Control and Prevention (CDC), 28–29, 41–43, 45, 47–48, 53–54, 134, 144–45, 180–81, 184–85, 187
Change4Life, 50
Child-like, 5, 8
Children, 6, 9, 27–29, 41–44, 46–55, 59–62, 65, 79, 83, 100, 134, 139, 142–43, 146–48, 151–53, 156–57, 165–67, 170, 175–76, 179–80, 183–85, 188–89
Cholesterol, 93–94, 117, 172, 180
Christy Girls, 5, 183
Clinical interview, 62
Communicable Disease Center, 53. *See also* Centers for Disease Control and Prevention (CDC)
Copenhagen City Heart Study, 129
Copenhagen General Population Study, 129
Coronary heart disease, 31, 112, 147
Correlation, 32–33, 73, 109, 133. *See also* Cause and effect
Corset, 5–6
Cortisol, 37. *See also* Epinephrine; Stress hormones
Cosmetic surgery, 15, 101. *See also* Plastic surgery
Crawford, Cindy, 12, 184

Death, 7, 19–20, 22, 33, 63, 80, 92, 116, 127–32, 166, 172. *See also* Lifespan

Department of Health and Human Services, United States (DHHS), 53
Depression, 60, 70, 81, 136. *See also* Mood disorders
Diabetes, 18, 20, 25–26, 32, 37, 53, 90, 110–15, 117–18, 122, 127–28, 131, 135, 139, 151, 173–74, 180
Diet. *See* Dieting
Diet and Health, with Key to the Calories, 7, 183. *See also* Peters, Lulu Hunt
Diet food, 12, 171, 184
Diethylpropion, 60. *See also* Bezphetamine; Phendimetrazine; Phentermine
Dietician, 69, 78, 92–93, 149, 167, 169, 174, 176
Dieting, 6–7, 12, 17, 19–20, 35–37, 52, 57–58, 61–62, 78, 84, 88–90, 92–95, 99, 103, 111, 120–21, 123–28, 155, 169–73, 175–76, 183–84, 188. *See also* Weight loss
Distress, 81, 84. *See also* Stress
Division of Nutrition, Physical Activity, and Obesity, 53. *See also* Centers for Disease Control and Prevention (CDC)
DNA, 113

Eating disorders, 12, 18–20, 26, 52, 88, 96, 156. *See also specific eating disorders*
Ectomorph, 15, 184. *See also* Endomorph; Mesomorph
1873 Comstock Law, 4
Endomorph, 15, 184. *See also* Ectomorph; Mesomorph
Epinephrine, 37. *See also* Cortisol; Stress hormones
Estrogen, 113

Exercise, 12, 17–19, 29, 35–37,
    57, 59, 61, 69, 76–77, 83,
    87–89, 103, 109, 111, 120–21,
    126–28, 138, 143, 158–59,
    168–74, 176, 188
Exercise is Medicine®, 188

Fashion, 4–10, 12, 18, 179–80. See
    also Fashion plate
Fashion plate, 4, 179
Fat. See Body fat
Fatty liver disease. See Nonalcoholic
    fatty liver disease
Feminine, 9, 11–12, 16
Fight or flight, 37
Fisher Girls, 5, 183
Fitness, 13–15, 55, 76–77, 101,
    155–56, 158–59, 165
Flapper, 5–6, 179, 183–84
Focusing illusion, 105–7, 179
Food and Drug Administration
    (FDA), 60

Gastric sleeve, 63
Gastrointestinal, 20, 61–63, 123
Genetics, 27, 32, 37, 58, 91, 102, 119,
    124, 133, 141, 177
Gibson, Charles, 4, 180. See also
    Gibson Girl
Gibson Girl, 4–5, 180, 183
Gilbert, Daniel, 105–6. See also
    Affective forecasting
Glucose, 83, 110–11, 172
Great War. See World War I
Growth charts, 27–29, 42, 180,
    183–85
Growth curve, 27–28, 184

Hackley, Madame E. Azalia, 7
Hair loss, 13–14
Hays Code of the 1930s, 8, 184
Health, 183–85, 187–88, 190; and ad
    campaigns, 49–51; and anti-fat
    bias, 67–68, 70–73, 75–76,
80–84; behavior management,
    58–59; and BMI, 21–40; and
    BMI report cards, 165–67; and
    cancer, 113; and costs of high
    BMI, 30–33, 134–37; definition
    of, 22; and dieting, 175–77;
    and disease, 110, 116–18; and
    growth charts, 27, 29; and
    happiness, 106; Health at Every
    Size®, 87–96, 149–61; and
    HIPAA, 180; and ideal body, 7,
    17–20, 99–100; and insurance,
    29, 34–35; and law, the,
    144–48; and life expectancy,
    129, 131–32; and long-term
    weight loss, 119, 122, 126–27;
    and measurement of, 23–24;
    and metabolic syndrome, 180;
    and nonalcoholic fatty liver
    disease, 114; and overweight
    or obese, 109–32; and personal
    responsibility, 138–41; and
    physically fit, being, 14–15;
    and political attitudes, 55; and
    prevention of obesity, 142–44;
    and public health policy,
    53–54; and school policies,
    52–53; weight gain, 168–70;
    and weight loss, 172–74; and
    weight loss surgery, 61–62,
    170–72
Health at Every Size® (HAES®),
    87–96, 149–61, 165, 167, 169,
    172, 174, 176–77, 185, 187,
    188, 189. See also Bacon, Linda
Health insurance, 24, 29–35, 80, 138,
    157, 180, 185
Health Insurance Portability and
    Accountability Act. See HIPAA
Held, Anna, 5
Hepburn, Audrey, 11, 194
Herbal supplements, 61
Hernia, 62–63, 172

Heroin chic, 12, 180, 185. *See also* Moss, Kate

HIPAA, 24, 180, 185

Hollywood, 15, 100

Hormones, 37, 111, 117

Hornesby, Lelie. *See* Twiggy

"Human Starvation and Its Consequences," 26, 184. *See also* Keys, Ancel

Hunger, 59, 61, 90, 150, 180

Hypercapnia, 113

Hyperglycemic, 111

Hypertension, 25, 112, 122, 127–28, 135

Hypoxia, 113

Impotence, 16

Income to poverty ratio, 47–48. *See also* Poverty threshold

"Indices of Relative Weight and Obesity," 26, 184. *See also* Keys, Ancel

Institute of Medicine, 52, 147

Insulin, 18, 110–11, 113–14, 118

Insurance. *See* Health insurance; Life insurance

Internalization, 17–18, 83–84

International Classification of Diseases (ICD), 25

Intra-abdominal fat, 117

Just-deserts responsibility, 140–41

Keys, Ancel, 26, 184. *See also* BMI; Quetelet Index

Ladies' Home Journal, 4, 183

Laparoscopic surgery, 62

Learned helplessness, 140

Let's Move!, 54, 156, 185, 188

Life insurance, 31, 133

Lifespan, 31, 143

Lorcaserin, 60

Low income, 47–48

Maine, Margo, 10. *See also* Barbie® doll

Makeup, 7–9

Malnutrition, 20

Masculinity, 13, 15–16

Mean, 38. *See also* Statistical average

Medical records, 27. *See also* HIPAA

Medication, 7, 18, 29, 57, 59–61, 72, 121, 123, 127, 172. *See also* Pharmacotherapy

Mental health, 3, 18–19, 22–23, 77, 81, 96, 100, 136–37, 140, 149–50, 169–70, 188

Mesomorph, 15, 184. *See also* Ectomorph; Endomorph

Metabolic syndrome, 95, 117–18, 128, 152, 174, 180

Metabolism, 36–37, 58, 61, 88–89, 110, 114. *See also* Basal metabolic rate

Monroe, Marilyn, 11, 184

Mood disorders, 70, 81. *See also* Depression

Moral hazard, 35

Morbidity, 22

Mortality rate, 19, 55, 64, 80, 127–31

Moss, Kate, 12, 180, 185

MRS degree, 10

Muscle dysmorphia, 19

Muscular ideal, 17–19, 36, 180. *See also* Body shape and size; Thin ideal

National Cancer Institute (NCI), 112–13

National Center for Health Statistics (NCHS), 27–28, 184. *See also* Growth charts

National Organization of Women (NOW), 11

National Weight Control Registry (NWCR), 120, 122

Negatively skewed distribution, 39. *See also* Positively

skewed distribution; Skewed distribution
Neurotransmitters, 60
1977 NCHS Growth Charts, 28, 184
Nineteenth Amendment, 4, 21
Nonalcoholic fatty liver disease, 114–15
Normal curve, 38–39
Normal distribution, 38–39

Obama, Michelle, 54, 156, 185, 188. See also *Let's Move!*
Obesity, 180, 185; and ad campaigns, 49–51, 185; and age, 42–43; and anti-fat bias, 65–66, 69–70, 72–73, 77–81, 85; and behavior management, 59; and BMI, 26, 30, 33, 35, 184; and BMI report cards, 166; and cancer, 112–13; and cardiovascular disease, 112; and CDC, 187; and costs, 132–37; and diabetes, 110–11; and education level, 48–49; and growth charts; and health, 109–18; and Health at Every Size®, 87, 90, 92, 94, 150, 153–57, 160; and income status, 46–48; and law, the, 144–48; and *Let's Move!*, 188; and life expectancy, 128–31; and long-term weight loss, 119, 124–25, 127; and medication therapy, 59; and nonalcoholic fatty liver disease, 114–15; and Obesity Action Coalition, 189; and osteoarthritis, 115–16; and personal choice, 133–48; and personal responsibility, 138–39, 141; and political attitudes towards, 54–56; and political attitudes towards, 54; and prevention efforts, 49–64, 141–44; and public health policy, 53–54; and questioning the research, 116–18; and race/ethnicity, 44–46; and rates of, 41–49; and Rudd Center for Food Policy and Obesity, 189; and school policies, 51–53; and sex, 43–44; and size discrimination, 56; and weight loss, 174; and weight loss surgery, 61–63, 171; and World Health Organization (WHO), 190. *See also* Overweight
Obsessive-compulsive disorder (OCD), 20
Off-label use, 60
Orlistat, 60
Osteopenia, 20
Osteoporosis, 20
Over-the-counter, 18, 29, 60–61
Overweight, 65, 133, 180–81, 183, 185; and access to services, 73; and ad campaigns, 49–51; and airlines, 74–75; and anti-fat bias, 67, 69–72; and behavior management, 59; and BMI, 26, 41; and BMI report cards, 165–66; and cardiovascular disease, 111; and costs, 31, 33, 35, 136; and diabetes, 110; and fitness and exercise facilities, 76–77; and growth charts, 28–29; and health, 109–32, 176; and Health at Every Size®, 95, 149–59; and ideal body, 12, 14–15; and internalization of weight stigma, 84; and law, the, 146; and life expectancy, 128–32; and long-term weight loss, 118–28; and medical care, 66, 77–78; and medication therapy, 59; and nonalcoholic fatty liver disease, 114; and normal (bell) curve, 39; and one-size-fits-all, dangers of, 72–73; and osteoarthritis;

and other services, 79; and
personal responsibility, 138–39;
and political attitudes towards,
54–56; and psychological effects,
80–81; and public health policy,
53; and school policies, 52; and
size discrimination, 56; and
weight gain, 168–69; and weight
loss, 173–74; and what should be
done, 141. *See also* Obesity
Oxygen, 113–14

Peters, Lulu Hunt, 7, 183. See also
*Diet and Health, with Key to the
Calories*
Phalloplasty, 16
Pharmacotherapy, 59. *See also*
Medication
Phendimetrazine, 60. *See also*
Bezphetamine; Diethylpropion;
Phentermine
Phentermine, 60. *See also*
Bezphetamine; Diethylpropion;
Phendimetrazine
Phentermine-topiramate, 60
Plastic surgery, 101. *See also*
Cosmetic surgery
Ponderal index, 26. *See also* BMI
Positively skewed distribution,
38–39. *See also* Negatively
skewed distribution; Skewed
distribution
Poverty threshold, 46–47. *See also*
Income to poverty ratio
Pre-bariatric surgery counseling, 61
Primary care provider (PCP), 29,
176, 180
Pro-thin bias, 66, 68
Psychological assessment, 62
Psychologist, licensed, 62, 149

Qsymia, 60
Quetelet, Adolphe, 25–26, 179, 183.
See also Quetelet Index

Quetelet Index, 25–26, 183–84. *See
also* BMI

Reverse causality, 130, 181
Roadmap for Health Measurement
and Accountability, The,
23–24, 185
Rosie the Riveter, 9
Roux-en-Y gastric bypass, 62–63

Satiety, 36, 61, 90, 180
Self-esteem, 12–13, 18, 50, 52, 70,
81, 88, 93–94, 100, 136,
152, 170
Serotonin, 60
Set point, 36
Sex symbol, 11
Sexual functioning, 13–14, 16
Sexuality, 4, 8, 16, 179, 184
Shirtwaist, 4–5
Showgirl, 5
Size discrimination, 56, 189. *See also*
Anti-fat bias
Skewed distribution, 38–40. *See also*
Negatively skewed distribution;
Positively skewed distribution
Skinny, 15, 17–18. *See also* Thin
Sleep apnea, 113–14
SnackRight, 50
Social marketing, 50–51
Statistical average, 38–39. *See
also* Mean
Steatosis, 114
*Stop Sugarcoating It,
Georgia*, 49, 51
Stress, 4, 37, 72, 80–81, 83, 91, 170.
See also Distress
Stress hormones, 37. *See also*
Cortisol; Epinephrine
Stroke, 111, 114, 117, 127, 130, 173,
180, 187
Stuart/Meredith Growth Charts, 27.
See also Growth charts
Subcutaneous fat, 117

Substance use disorders, 20, 60, 80–81
Suffragists, 3, 5
Sympathetic nervous system, 37

Take-charge responsibility, 140
Thin, 3, 6–7, 11, 18, 52, 67–68, 73, 76–77, 80, 89, 92, 107, 110, 119, 168, 171. *See also* Skinny; Thinner; Thinness
Thin ideal, 17–19, 36, 100, 181. *See also* Body shape and size
Thinner, 6–7, 18, 66–67, 73, 110, 150, 175. *See also* Skinny; Thin; Thinness
Thinness, 56, 75, 109. *See also* Skinny; Thin; Thinner
Triglycerides, 59, 117, 172, 180
Twiggy, 11, 184
Type 1 diabetes, 111. *See also* Diabetes; Type 2 diabetes
Type 2 diabetes, 110–11, 113. *See also* Diabetes; Type 1 diabetes

U.S. Equal Employment Opportunity Commission (EEOC), 56

VERB, 50
Vertical sleeve gastrectomy (VSG), 62–63
Visceral fat, 117

Weight bias, 56–57, 69, 73, 79, 84, 189
Weight cycling, 17, 37, 58, 78, 122, 127. *See also* Yo-yo dieting
Weight discrimination, 56, 80–81, 188
Weight gain, 17, 35, 37, 39, 52–53, 57–58, 61, 63, 82, 87, 89, 93, 95–96, 113, 118–19,

123–24, 126–27, 136, 142, 144, 171, 179
Weight loss, 173–75, 184; and anti-fat bias, 72–73, 77, 80, 82; and beauty industry, 101; and behavior management, 57–59; and BMI, 26, 29–30, 34–37; and BMI report cards, 166–67 and cancer, 113; and happiness, 99, 106; and health, 109, 116, 176–77; and Health at Every Size®, 87–94, 150, 152–55, 157–59, 188; and ideal body, 7, 11–12, 17–18, 20; and law, the, 146; and life-expectancy, 130; long-term, 118–28; and medication therapy, 59–61; and personal responsibility, 131–42, 144; and public health policy, 53; and weight loss surgery, 63–64, 170–72, 179. *See also* Dieting
Weight loss surgery, 29, 57, 59, 61, 121, 170–72, 179. *See also* Bariatric surgery; *and specific types of weight loss surgeries*
Weight stigma, 65, 70, 72–73, 79, 81–84, 87
Weight Watchers®, 11, 58
World Health Organization (WHO), 22, 128–29, 134, 180–81, 184, 190
World War I, 5–6
World War II, 8–9, 26

Xenical, 60

YouBeauty.com Body Image Survey, 104
Yo-yo dieting, 17, 20, 37, 78, 89, 94, 124, 127, 169, 171–72. *See also* Weight cycling

About the Author

Christine L. B. Selby, PhD, is an associate professor of psychology at Husson University in Bangor, Maine, where she teaches introductory and upper-level psychology courses including a specialized course on eating disorders. Dr. Selby also maintains a part-time private practice as a licensed psychologist where she specializes in sport psychology and eating disorders. She is a member of the American Psychological Association (APA), the Academy for Eating Disorders, the International Association of Eating Disorder Professionals, the Association for Size Diversity and Health, and the Association for Applied Sport Psychology (AASP). As an active member of AASP, she cofounded and cochaired the Eating Disorder Special Interest Group. She was also president of the Society for Sport, Exercise & Performance Psychology (formerly known as the Division of Sport and Exercise Psychology). Dr. Selby is a certified eating disorder specialist, and certified consultant with AASP. She has presented nationally on topics primarily related to eating disorders in athletes and has published articles and book chapters in the area of eating disorders and related concerns in athletes. She is also the author of Greenwood's *Chilling Out: The Psychology of Relaxation.*